# PRAISE FOR *JUST BE WELL*

"If I had a complex, chronic illness, I would want a guide like Dr. Sult. I trust his deep intelligence and intuition, and I love his sense of humor. And Dr. Sult calls it as he sees it. In *Just Be Well*, Dr. Sult takes what can seem complicated and onerous—articulating the underlying causes of disease and what to do about it—and turns it into an accessible, captivating, and hope-filled read, complete with patient stories and his own personal journey of discovery. This book will provide direction for patients who are spinning their wheels in the dominant medical paradigm. It will also inspire physicians mired in the limitations of the same medical paradigm eager for a more effective approach."

**Kara N. Fitzgerald, ND**
Integrative and Functional Medicine
Co-author and editor, *Case Studies in Integrative and Functional Medicine*
Contributing author, *Textbook of Functional Medicine*
Contributing author, *Laboratory Evaluations for Integrative and Functional Medicine*

●-●-●

"This book was so much fun to read! It reminded me of the pleasure I experienced when reading Rachel Remen's *Kitchen Table Wisdom*. Not only did I learn a tremendous amount, but like reading a novel, I enjoyed the experience of story. Tom Sult is a master storyteller.

"Dr. Sult's book shows us why the medical profession must switch from concern about *what* a patient has (the diagnosis) to *why* they have it. In acute illness and injury, the diagnosis and appropriate protocol for treatment is important. In chronic illness, Dr. Sult helps us understand why it is time to say goodbye to the diagnosis. Instead, we must begin to figure out *why* the person has this problem at this time and how it relates to other problems she or he has. What is the underlying biochemistry? What is this person's past and present environment? What are this person's stressors and mindset?

"This book is the best explanation of functional medicine that I have ever read, and if we hope to reverse the upward trend of chronic disease in America, this book has the answers. I highly recommend it."

**Bill Manahan, MD**
Past president, American Holistic Medical Association

"Dr. Sult's opening question says it all: 'When was the last time you were completely and truly well?' If your answer is anything other than 'Today,' you need this book. An excellent introduction to functional medicine with great patient examples to illustrate all the key principles."

**Dr. Joseph Pizzorno, ND**
Editor-in-Chief, *Integrative Medicine, A Clinician's Journal*
Co-author, *Encyclopedia of Natural Medicine*
Vice-Chair, Board of the Institute for Functional Medicine

<br>

"Dr. Tom Sult is a trained believer, not just a writer of books. He has been there and understands the journey his patients have been on. The personal stories resonate and are instructive and easy to understand. Tom has captured the essence of functional medicine and distinguished it from our present broken system heading for economic disaster. *Just Be Well* is desperately needed, and it will have you reading until you finish it. As Socrates was told at the Oracle of Delphi: 'That which I do not know, I know that I do not know.' We are all in search of that wisdom."

**Mark Houston, MD, MS, MSc, FACP, FAHA, FASH, FACN**
Associate Clinical Professor of Medicine
Vanderbilt University School of Medicine
Director, Hypertension Insititute
Saint Thomas Hospital
Nashville, TN

<br>

"You are going to learn a lot from this book; that's true of many books. You are going to be *delighted* by this book; that's rarely true of any book. Dr. Sult has put together a narrative that tells the story of his lifelong pursuit of understanding the foundations of health and illnesses. When he says, 'Neither information nor knowledge is adequate; one must have wisdom to make impactful lasting change,' he's telling the truth. We can do without pleasure, but wisdom illuminated by the candle of delight . . . you simply cannot have too much. Enjoy!"

**David S. Jones, MD**
President, Institute for Functional Medicine

"From a leader in functional medicine, *Just Be Well* is an invitation to viewing your wellness as more than the absence of disease. Dr. Sult concisely creates a roadmap for a journey from illness and disease to optimal wellness."

**Joseph Lamb, MD**
Director of Intramural Clinical Research
MetaProteomics, LLC; Metagenics, Inc

"Once I started reading *Just Be Well*, I had a hard time putting it down. This is one of the most thoughtfully written non-fiction books by a doctor-writer that I have read in a long time. It is filled with fascinating stories that have changed the way I think about the practice of medicine. Sult clearly connects with his patients and writes from the heart, with a sharp eye for the art of being a physician. He has wisdom and a clarity that remind me of Atul Gawande."

**David Riley, MD**
Editor-in-Chief, *Global Advances in Health and Medicine*

"This book embodies all of the essential qualities of Dr. Tom Sult. The style is inquisitive, boldly honest, and full of intelligence, heart, and humor. His use of story and metaphor breathe life into concepts that are otherwise difficult to explain, and the chapters at times read like a detective novel; you can't wait to see what he will discover next! His examples of patients experiencing common problems for which he identifies uncommonly recognized causes bring hope to anyone with chronic medical conditions. After reading this book, you will want to find yourself a functional medicine doctor and participate in the movement to make medicine more personalized and patient focused. It's Dr. Sult's grateful tribute to those who have inspired him, and you, too, will be inspired by his words. If you can't have Dr. Sult as your doctor, at least you will benefit from his wisdom and experience in this fascinating exploration of functional medicine."

**Nancy Sudak, MD**
Executive Director, American Board of Integrative Holistic Medicine

# JUST BE WELL

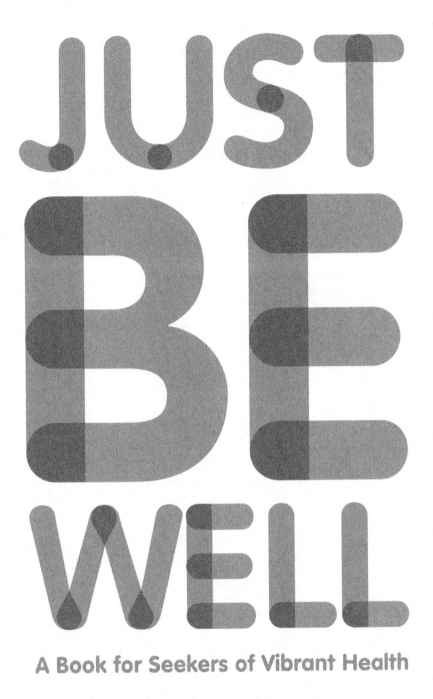

# JUST BE WELL

A Book for Seekers of Vibrant Health

Thomas A. Sult, MD

# JUST BE WELL

Writers of the Round Table Press
PO Box 511, Highland Park, IL 60035
www.roundtablecompanies.com

Publisher and Executive Editor: *Corey Michael Blake*
Executive Editor: *Katie Gutierrez*
Staff Editor: *Aaron Hierholzer*
Creative Director: *David Charles Cohen*
Directoress of Happiness: *Erin Cohen*
Director of Author Services: *Kristin Westberg*
Facts Keeper: *Mike Winicour*
Cover Design: *Analee Paz*
Interior Design and Layout: *Sunny DiMartino*
Proofreading: *Rita Hess*
Last Looks: *Sunny DiMartino*
Digital Conversion and Distribution: *Sunny DiMartino*

Printed in the United States of America

First Edition: September 2013
10  9  8  7  6  5  4  3  2

*Library of Congress Cataloging-in-Publication Data*
Sult, Thomas A.
Just be well: a book for seekers of vibrant health /
Thomas A. Sult, MD.—1st ed. p. cm.
ISBN Hardcover: 978-1-939418-39-5
ISBN Paperback: 978-1-939418-38-8
ISBN Digital: 978-1-939418-40-1
Library of Congress Control Number: 2013946842

RTC Publishing is an imprint of Writers of the Round Table, Inc.
Writers of the Round Table Press and the RTC Publishing logo
are trademarks of Writers of the Round Table, Inc.

# CONTENTS

*To my wife, Robin, for teaching me happiness.*

*To my boys, Andrew and John, for teaching me joy.*

*To Jackson, my first and as yet only grandchild, for teaching me wonder.*

*To my mother, Mary Ellen (a.k.a. Jane or Stan); my father, Arnell (a.k.a. Stormy); my brothers, Stan (who thought his name was a girl's name because of my mom's nickname) and Mike (who is the only one in the family with one name); and my sisters, Kathy (who was named after my Aunt Jimmy) and Cindy (who preferred to be called Cynthia in her youth): from you all I learned that love is infinite and unconditional, if not always tranquil. (My family's proclivity for having many strange additional names may also be the topic of my next book.)*

*And finally, to my patients, for showing me how to be a better doctor.*

# FOREWORD

You will learn a lot from this book; that's true of many books. You will be *delighted* by this book; that's rarely true of any book.

In *Just Be Well*, Dr. Tom Sult has put together a narrative that tells the story of his lifelong pursuit to understand the foundations of health and illnesses. When he says: "Neither information nor knowledge is adequate; one must have wisdom to make impactful lasting change," he's telling the truth.

Dr. Sult has a distinct style that allows his brilliance as a thinker and as a compassionate and sharing human being to shine through. I am delighted as I read his work; it sparkles. He started out to write a book that would explain his practice of functional medicine, a "how and why" text for his patients. With urging from those who read early drafts, he has extended his intention for a wider audience.

When I was asked to read his first draft, as I often am because of my 40-year association with the development of functional medicine through the Institute for Functional Medicine, I wrote back: "Tom, I think that you are on to something important by letting yourself express how it really, really is for you as a doctor and the journey that brings you to this place of wisdom." The wholeness of Tom, a person who is a physician, jumps out of the pages of this short book.

In *Just Be Well* Dr. Sult illustrates what functional medicine, a systems medicine approach to chronic illnesses, can mean and do for patients in the exam rooms of clinical medicine. Using and understanding the fundamental organizational and physiological processes within each of us as key nodes of biological influence allows doctors to find the underlying causes of disease. When properly in balance, these processes yield wellness; when out of balance, our body's systems devolve into dysfunction and disease. Through a robust and disciplined process of inquiry, we can discover the underlying causes of patients' illnesses.

Without this understanding and method of inquiry, compassionate physicians and suffering patients are offered but one treatment option in conventional medical practices: suppress symptoms and pain with pharmacological agents. However, empowered by knowledge of the active mechanisms and causes of illnesses, the physician and patient can work as a team to restore balance and health. Realigning a biological system that has spiraled into wobbling imbalance is the real trench work of the therapeutic partnership between physician and patient. Together, they can plan a different kind of medical intervention, taking aim on restoring equipoise. By marrying an understanding of the underlying physiological processes with an understanding of the environmental lifestyle determinants that have evoked the dysfunction, health can be restored.

In *Just Be Well*, Dr. Sult has taken a risk; he had initial reservations and worry that his early chapters might read like a *Pilgrim's Progress* travelogue of how a person develops into a doctor. I understand his concern, because in this book, Dr. Sult does not hide behind the usual cover of the physician's white coat. Instead, he candidly reveals his concern and love affair with his patients and his profession. I wrote to him in the initial stages of his book: "I hope that you will allow me to read on as your chapters continue to tumble out of you. I love the recurrent theme in your writing that shines through in sentences like this: *"It was another one of those moments—like my arrival in Grenada—where I looked at the scene before me, smiled, and thought, I am home."*

When Dr. Sult finished this book, I wrote again with congratulations: "We can do without pleasure, but wisdom illuminated by the candle of delight—we simply cannot have too much of either." My hope is that *Just Be Well* finds a wide readership. Those readers lucky enough to come in contact with this book will be both informed and delighted by their experience.

—*David S. Jones, MD*
*President, Institute for Functional Medicine*

# ACKNOWLEDGMENTS

I grew up in a magical time in a magical place: the 1960s and '70s in what is now called Silicon Valley. It was a time and place where anything was possible. My older brother went to high school with a guy named Steve Jobs. My dad, who worked at the cutting edge of computers, was a ham radio operator, so we always had interesting stuff like microphones, speakers, amplifiers, and solar cells around the house or were talking to someone in Australia or wherever on the radio. My mom was the family's glue, ever present at school events and activities.

As the fourth of five kids, I had a lot of freedom. My parents were no longer paralyzed with fear about me falling on my head—after all, none of my older siblings had—so I could explore my curiosities until I gave my parents reason to reign me back in. Generally speaking, I had absolute autonomy. I was able to go rock climbing both at the local crags and in the High Sierra in Yosemite. I became an assistant guide at the wilderness center and eventually a mountain guide.

Like my brother (and Steve Jobs), I attended Homestead High School. I wasn't a great student, but I was given a great opportunity and had many wonderful teachers who taught many great classes (the most important to me was "Situation Ethics"—an introduction to philosophy and many different worldviews). Thank you.

At DeAnza Junior College, a counselor told me that with my grades, medical school was not a realistic choice. Many years later, I sent him a copy of my diploma from UCLA School of Medicine . . . I had scrawled across it in red: "Fuck you." I am sure he looked at it in complete bafflement and would never remember me now. But he motivated me. So, thanks.

No book is written in isolation. This book is the cumulative wisdom of all of my many teachers. Jeff Bland, PhD, is the "father" of functional medicine. He, along with many fellow teachers at the Institute for Functional Medicine, shaped my thinking and ideas . . . ideas discussed late into the night, lubricated by fellowship and perhaps a bit of spirits, both liquid and ethereal. You can read more about my amazing colleagues at the Institute here: www.functional medicine.org/about/ourteam/faculty.

On my first day of college, I was excused from English 101 to be moved to English for Boneheads. If not for the wonderful assistance of Katie Gutierrez, my "Penmaster General," this work would be largely unintelligible. Thanks also to the rest of the team at Round Table Companies, Inc. for assistance in all aspects of this work, from punctuation to personal growth.

There are undoubtedly many others to whom I am deeply indebted. To those of you whom I have not mentioned, I am sorry for the omission but remain deeply grateful to you.

# INTRODUCTION

When was the last time you were completely and truly well? I don't mean the last time you "felt okay" for a day or two; I mean *completely well*.

This is not an easy question to answer. In part, it's because "completely well" is a nebulous term. It's different for everyone and yours to define. What I am really asking is this: when did your health change? What was the year, the month, the moment that your health shifted from completely well—whatever that means for you—to what it is now? The answer is crucial, because knowing *when* your health changed means we can explore the most important question of all: *why?*

If you are like most patients I see, you have been suffering from chronic illness for longer than you care to recall. You're a regular with your local doctor, have been referred to one or more specialists, and have traveled to universities and/or the Mayo Clinic in an effort to determine *what* is wrong with your health. You've been given a variety of diagnoses, with a drug to combat each symptom and further drugs to counteract the side effects of the first batch. You are anxious because you are ill and ill because you are anxious. Despite all your efforts, all the doctors' visits, research, and medication—a devastatingly frustrating cycle—the problems persist. At some point, not only did the doctors start to doubt you, but you also started to doubt yourself.

Whether you have found this book through research, a recommendation, or a doctor, you are probably feeling desperate. But you are not defeated. Functional medicine can restore hope. Functional medicine can unleash your awesome capacity to heal.

What many people don't understand is that disease is the body doing what it is supposed to do, given its environment. If the body is placed in a toxic environment, it will fiercely try to detoxify. If the body is given an inflammatory diet, it will fiercely try to manage that inflammation. Unfortunately, the body has only a finite capacity for trying to restore balance. If you're living an inflammatory lifestyle (fast food, little sleep), you are overriding its abilities. At this point, it's not enough to tell you *what* you have and hand you a prescription. Rather, functional medicine is going to try to restore balance to your total lifestyle. And lifestyle balance isn't just an add-on—it has been shown that genetics is only about 30 percent of the problem. Seventy percent of our health is related to lifestyle, diet, and environment. If there's a mismatch between our genetics and our environment, disease will result—often chronic, complex disease. Functional medicine is about trying to understand, identify, and optimize lifestyle factors to rebalance genes with lifestyle and environmental factors.

So, how do we restore balance? By asking *why*. *Why* do you have, for example, inflammation? What is happening with your personal underlying biochemistry? Is there a defect in the way your body methylates? A problem with how you process fatty acids? Do you have too robust an ability to produce inflammatory chemicals? We ask the question "Why?" in an inquisitive way rather than a deterministic way. The ultimate answer is often unknowable, but the inquisitive nature of the question allows us to explore new opportunities. For example, if you are diagnosed with fibromyalgia, there are only a select number of treatments available. They may include pain management strategies, medications, and—if you're seeing a holistic provider—perhaps diet and lifestyle modifications and acupuncture. But asking the fundamentally different question "*Why* might I have fibromyalgia?" and exploring the disease's potential causes in your underlying physiology may lead to new understanding and fundamentally different areas of intervention. In other words, whatever the answers are, by understanding *why*, we can move forward into *how*—how to go from dis-ease to ease.

*How* varies. What I can tell you is this: there is no quick fix. It's not about Prozac or St. John's Wort, steroidal injections, or fish oil; functional medicine is neither conventional medicine nor green pharmacy ("green pharmacy" simply refers to treatment with herbs or vitamins in place of pharmaceutical medicines). Instead, I call it *audience participation medicine*. You've come to a theater where the actors assume you are part of their play. Collaboration isn't just important to a successful outcome; it's essential.

Functional medicine does not divide disease up by organ system (as traditional medicine does) but instead addresses the underlying physiological process that is contributing to a patient's condition. Functional medicine addresses eight of these processes, each of which comprises an area of the functional medicine "matrix" that you'll learn about in the following chapters. The core content of this book covers each of these eight areas in a separate chapter, with a case study that has been carefully selected to illustrate how that area works. However, it's important to keep in mind that, generally speaking, people have difficulty in multiple areas of the matrix. Throughout this book, I'll reemphasize the interconnected nature of human health and of the matrix, but I feel the need to establish at the outset that when it comes to functional medicine, virtually nothing happens in isolation.

Consider this book, then, your introduction to audience participation medicine. You will learn about:

- The differences between conventional care and functional medicine
- The differences between green pharmacy and functional medicine
- Using the "three-legged stool" consisting of the timeline, the story, and the matrix to define a treatment plan
- Clinical imbalances as found on the functional medicine matrix
- How imbalances in one area can create symptoms in another, seemingly unrelated area
- The power of understanding your "story"
- Common treatments for imbalances
- How functional medicine can transform not just bodily health but also mental and spiritual well-being

While this book will help you understand the power of the journey you're taking, it is only the tip of the iceberg. Each chapter can significantly help you optimize wellness, but it's only the precursor to what can be achieved by partnering with a functional medicine doctor. After all, no book, no matter how good, can replace the power of a doctor asking *why* . . . and listening for the answer. So often, people come to me with a book—a wonderful book—about health. But the book is, by definition, general. Functional medicine is personalized. My goal is that this book will start you down the path of personalized care. You'll read about many of my patients who've made great strides back toward health, and you'll learn, through self-exploration, how you can start your own journey. At the very least, this book will help you understand what your functional medicine doctor is trying to do and how you can help him.

Finally, remember: this book **is not about disease**. Neither is functional medicine. Rather, it is about optimizing wellness. When we optimize wellness, there is no room for disease. There is only, once again, the chance to just be well.

—*Thomas A. Sult, MD*

# Chapter 1

# THE PURPOSE OF A DOCTOR

Most patients I see have been through the wringer. After an extensive, multi-physician, multi-specialty workup that costs thousands of dollars, they are left with inconclusive, conflicting, or confusing results. One supposedly firm diagnosis leads to another, sending the patient reeling through a maze of new physicians, medications, and side effects. The original diagnosis often is replaced, leaving patients with a medicine cabinet full of pills and a huge question mark about their health and future. Worse yet, many are told it's all in their head. By the time they end up in my office, all the conventional, standard, run-of-the-mill stuff has already been done—twice. We have to start looking elsewhere. But why? Haven't the other specialists already done that?

The previous doctors, whether primary care doctors, local or regional specialists, or ultra-specialists from a university or the Mayo Clinic, have all been asking the same basic set of questions to achieve the same goal: to find a disease. A practitioner of functional medicine, on the other hand, asks fundamentally different questions. While the other doctors ask *what*, we functional medicine doctors ask *why*. *Why* do you have this illness? *How* are you different?

These questions are designed to identify what we call antecedents, triggers, and mediators. Antecedents are those things, often genetic, that may predispose you to an illness. If you dig deep and look hard enough, most people with a chronic illness can identify an event or a time when things seemed to go haywire. That is the trigger. Mediators are what keep the illness going. To help us figure out what these factors are in a patient, we ask questions that greatly differ from those a regular physician would ask. One of the most important is this one: when was the last time you were truly well—not for a day or two but *truly, truly* well? These fundamentally different questions lead to profoundly different answers from the patient—and to profoundly different ways of treating illness. They help us understand when wellness started to fade away and how we can restore it.

Some people have suggested that wellness is the absence of disease. We functional medicine doctors know that this is a flawed idea, because wellness is a vibrant state of well-being—not just the absence of sickness. However, the opposite of this is true: disease can only exist in the absence of wellness. The questions we ask help us find the imbalances that have led a person from a place of ease to a place of dis-ease. Understanding that path can help us lead the patient back to his or her place of wellness.

So, when people ask, "Haven't the other specialists already done this?" my answer is always an emphatic no.

●-●-●

When I first began questioning what the "authorities" said, it was out of necessity. I wasn't a good student, and I was told many times that I couldn't read and wouldn't amount to anything. But the people who told me those things weren't right—they simply hadn't asked *why* I performed the way I did.

On the last day of third grade, kids around me were giddy with the anticipation of summer in Cupertino, California. We had just been handed our report cards, and most were sharing their grades with everyone else. But my face turned ashen when I opened mine—the paper held mostly Fs and a note that I'd have to repeat the grade. I thought of the year that had passed—the struggle to find key words in a text I could use to understand the reading, the red-penned tests that I crumpled into my lunch box, the overwhelming feeling of inferiority—and wanted to cry at the thought of doing it all again. When I slinked dejectedly into the house, my mom told me she already knew about my grades. She'd talked to the teachers and decided to let me find out on my own.

That summer, I was diagnosed with what was then called "minimal brain dysfunction"—a label for a condition we now know as dyslexia. I didn't know what it meant, but I believed I was stupid because I couldn't read as well as my peers.

Years later, in college, I found that I could actually tutor my peers in concepts I fully understood and they did not. After tests, they would tell me, "I wouldn't have gotten this A without you"—and yet I was still making Bs. Dyslexia impaired my test-taking skills, and my thinking process was more random than linear. While a linear-minded person is tied to logical associations and sequential progressions, people like me can hold many ideas—sometimes even conflicting ones—in their minds at the same time. (Author and medical doctor Blake Charlton pointed to recent studies and functional MRIs that demonstrate a range of *abilities* people with dyslexia have, including excellent three-dimensional and spatial reasoning[1]). If you don't view the world in a linear, sequential way, you will likely have a great deal of difficulty in a conventional school; most school teachers are attracted to their profession because they see this sort of logical progression as knowledge. But a study of major scientific discoveries reveals that most were the result of nonlinear moments of inspiration and deeply intuitive insights rather than lock-step linear progression.

Because I was starting to understand this, I began shedding the idea that I was just dumber than everyone around me was. As an undergraduate, I started as a fine arts (photography) major but later switched to chemistry, and in a chemistry class at Chico State, the professor gave me some reinforcement I never forgot. "You can compete with those guys," he told me. "Don't even think about it—whatever you want to do, do it." So I decided to try for medical school—a lifelong dream, despite my dyslexia.

In 1981, I applied to forty-two medical schools in the United States. My science GPA was a 3.5, and my overall GPA was a 3.0. I didn't think that was so terrible, but I didn't get a single interview. I was crushed (though I did find out later that friends of mine with 4.0 GPAs couldn't even get into *their* top three schools).

After that rejection, I started to think I wasn't cut out for an academic career. Nevertheless, I decided I'd apply again the next year. In the meantime, I continued a job I'd taken as a paramedic and also continued my work as a mountain guide.

---

1   Charlton, Blake, "Defining My Dyslexia." *The New York Times*, May 23, 2013. Accessed July 4, 2013, http://www.nytimes.com/2013/05/23/opinion/defining-my-own-dyslexia.html?_r=0.

Initially, life as a paramedic was fulfilling. I appreciated its hands-on nature. Soon, though, I began finding the protocol-driven structure of the work tiring. After inserting a certain number of IVs and endotracheal tubes, it's just not that exciting anymore. Even with the worst trauma case, there was no chance of solving a puzzle or answering a tough question. It was mostly protocol. Before the doctor even arrived, I had already ordered the appropriate labs and called in all the various teams—the x-ray people, the operating room team, and so on. The mystery was gone. And again, I realized I wasn't dumb after all: I often arrived at a patient's diagnosis as quickly as the ER doctor did.

My second round of medical school applications went just like my first. With forty-two more rejection letters on my hands, I started wondering what the hell I was going to do with my life. Medical school seemed to be slipping further from my realistic possibilities. And yet, I wasn't ready to give up.

My next move was to San Francisco and into a field that, at the time, was gaining more and more visibility: acupuncture. Its practitioners were just becoming recognized and licensed, and it seemed like something I could do. Acupuncture school surrounded me with a variety of people. Of my twenty-five classmates, some were students like me who hadn't gotten into medical school, others were physicians who'd decided to change specialties, and a few hardcore hippie-dippy types added interest. I didn't know it yet, but acupuncture school was my initial step toward holistic medicine.

At first, the vocabulary of acupuncture was totally foreign to me, and it was a steep learning curve to figure out what my teachers were talking about. They lectured about the "five elements," the *yin* and the *yang*, all these Eastern philosophical terms. And when they talked about the liver, for example, they weren't referring to that organ in the upper right quadrant of the abdomen but the energetic connections all over the body that encompass the liver meridian.

I found that acupuncture school was the perfect place to exercise suspending judgment. In my classes, I let the information wash over me and tried to accept it for what it was rather than immediately criticize it. This felt like a natural extension of my nonlinear learning style. For once, my way of looking at the world was a strength. School was exciting, energizing, and interesting. I felt as if I were on a quest.

The most important idea I took from acupuncture was the idea of interconnectedness at every level. The classic example is Dizzy Dean, the 1930s baseball player who pitched for the St. Louis Cardinals, the Chicago Cubs, and the St. Louis Browns. In the 1937 All-Star game, a line drive nailed Dean on the big toe, instantly fracturing it. ("Fractured?" Dean said after the diagnosis. "Hell, the damn thing's broken!") He went back to the game too soon, his toe hurting so badly he changed his windup and delivery to avoid landing on it as hard. Over the next several weeks, he developed an injury in his shoulder as a result of the different motion. One year later, the man once known as baseball's greatest pitcher was just another guy throwing a ball. Three years after that, his career was over.

The story shows the pervasive connectedness of the human body: two seemingly disparate body parts—toe and shoulder—are actually linked through gait, habitus, and biomechanics. But the connections go deeper than the framework of the body: we know, for example, that blood sugar is related to insulin, insulin is related to cortisol, cortisol is related to osteoporosis, and on and on. When one link in the chain is off, the whole system becomes distorted. In fact, many chronic diseases are simply the body's attempt at rebalancing given the new distorted physiology. When you take that into consideration, you start to understand that the treatment of the disease is less about the disease itself and more about resolving the original distortion.

At acupuncture school, I still thought I would apply to medical school a third time. Some of my peers were talking about foreign medical schools, but I rejected the idea at first. If those schools were any good, why hadn't my professors mentioned them? The truth was that back then, as today, most professors and physicians looked down upon foreign medical schools. (Around this time, the state of New York was debating whether to certify out-of-country schools, and the dean of Cambridge's medical school pointed out the absurdity of this attitude: "We've been around an awful lot longer than you have," he said, "so maybe we should be certifying *your* medical schools.")

When I found out that a foreign school was a viable option and that I had a good chance of getting in, I decided to apply for a program in the Caribbean island of Grenada. After an interview at a hotel in Santa Monica, I learned I'd been accepted. I wept when I got the news. It had been a long and difficult journey, but in 1982, I was off to my first year at St. George's University Medical School.

I spent two years in Grenada, and I loved every second of it. The foreignness, the chaos—even the sense of danger—excited me. When I first got off the plane, I was confronted by a giant poster of Maurice Bishop (the prime minister of Grenada), Fidel Castro, and Daniel Ortega; it proclaimed them the three giants of socialism. The man who checked my passport stood not behind a glass wall but behind chicken wire, and no one seemed bothered by the guys walking around with machine guns. I'd been to third-world countries before, and I instantly knew that Grenada was where I wanted to be.

Outside the airport, where people were being dropped off and picked up, it was complete bedlam. Dozens of busses waited to collect tourists, and eager drivers grabbed the luggage out of your hand in an effort to lead you to their vehicles. Vans meant to hold nine were stuffed with nearly twenty people. Everyone seemed to be screaming at me. I looked at the mayhem, the complete sensory overload, and smiled. *This is fantastic*, I thought. *This is home.* (Soon, things would become even more chaotic, with President Reagan's invasion of Grenada in 1983. I was there when it happened—but perhaps that's the subject of another book.)

Going on rounds at Saint George's Hospital was like visiting a Civil War battle ward. There were no glass windows, just screens, and no kitchen. If you were sick and your family didn't bring you food, you didn't eat. The wards were open, like the set of a 1940s movie. Because there wasn't much technology (e.g., x-rays, CTs), there was tremendous importance placed on the physical diagnosis. Most of the physicians in Grenada had been trained in England, and the English system emphasizes physical diagnosis, so I was lucky to be trained by excellent physical diagnosticians.

Without access to equipment, we had to understand heart sounds in a very deep way. The doctor took his stethoscope and rested it on five or six different places on the patient's chest, listening intently to each sound. Based only on that, he came up with a diagnosis—"You have mitral stenosis." In contrast, you'd get one quick listen in today's U.S. emergency room and be sent off for an echocardiogram for a definitive diagnosis. That's not to denigrate the physician doing this—it's irrelevant to listen so intensely to a heartbeat when machines nearby can arguably do the job more effectively. But the experience of working so intimately with patients changed my conception of how doctors and patients interact. I was used to doctors saying things like "Sounds like there's something going on with your heart; we're going to get an echocardiogram" (and how terrifying is that?), but now I saw that they could say, "Well, Mrs. Jones, I just listened to your heart very carefully, and it appears that you have a condition known as mitral stenosis. I don't think it's serious because of the way it sounds, but to be sure, we're going to get an echocardiogram." The action—sending the patient for an echocardiogram—is the same, but the *inter*action is very different. One does not take the patient's emotional response into account; the other does.

Despite forcing me to learn to operate without high technology, St. George's medical program was typical of modern medicine in that it was hyper-reductionist. Problems in patients were looked at on a very small scale; there was little examination of the whole-body system and how it may be affecting the problem. There was no focus on the Dizzy Dean style of interconnectedness that I'd seen so clearly in acupuncture school. However, another aspect of my education on Grenada helped fill that gap.

In my second semester, I moved off campus and into the basement of a family that, by Grenadian standards, lived a high-class life. (By our modern American standards, they would have been middle class.) This family was always hosting gatherings of family and friends and engaging in thoughtful conversations about politics, culture, and Grenada's place in the world. Through them, I met two "bush doctors"—local herbalists and shamans. Contrary to what I may have thought a year earlier, they didn't wear grass skirts; they walked around in normal clothes. But one of them did razz me about being in medical school. To him, getting a medical degree was tantamount to being a technician. If I wanted to be a real healer, he said, I needed to apprentice with a bush doctor. I suspended judgment and listened to him.

The bush doctors' work was fascinating, and I started being invited to people's houses to participate not just in herbal remedies but also in spiritual ceremonies. They used trance states, chants, prayer, and occasionally psychoactive herbs to affect health through the spirit world.

One evening after dinner, and well after dark (sunset is very early at ten degrees north latitude), I walked with a healer from the house I was staying in to the home of a family that lived in one of the shanties dotting Granada's walking paths. Their home was a simple structure, one ten-foot by ten-foot room that housed two adults and four or five kids. One of the children, a young girl, had a bad case of what looked like the flu. The child was lying on a mat on the floor. She had a high fever with hallucinations and chills, and she was sweating and shaking so badly that her mother was convinced she was possessed.

The healer put his hand on the girl and said an incantation I didn't understand. Then he mixed a complex anti-fever herbal medicine for the girl—pinches of this and that from his collection of bags, ground up with a mortar and pestle and made into a tea. We stayed for nearly two more hours, talking to the family and watching over the girl. By the time we left, her fever had broken. The mother was convinced she'd just witnessed a miracle. She had gone from streaming tears of fear to streaming tears of joy. She truly believed this healer had cast the devil out of her daughter. The healer told the mother that this was not the devil—just a misguided spirit. He explained to her that he had helped the spirit find his way home and that he would no longer be bothering her child. He also explained that the herbs would keep the girl's fever under control for the next several days while she healed. As we walked back, I questioned him about his belief in the spirit world. He sensed my skepticism, patted me on the back—a parental gesture to show he wasn't just blowing me off but instead understood my lack of belief—and assured me that such things do exist.

I found in the bush doctors a more holistic approach that took into account the person's total being, an approach more aligned with the interconnectedness I'd seen in acupuncture school. Throughout the rest of my two years of formal medical school in Grenada, I took the educational piece for what it was—an approximation of reality—and did my best to put the information I was learning into a larger context of connectedness rather than just cramming facts in my brain. I didn't see the reductionist approach as a conflict as much as a small piece of a very large puzzle. In class, I'd think, *I'm learning about what the liver does in isolation. But the liver has to exist in a larger context.*

Being immersed in the culture of Grenada for two years made me rethink how I viewed the world. On a trip home to California, I was shocked at the contrast in grocery stores—these stores had more types of dog food than those in Grenada had of total *human* food. I saw how deeply and unnecessarily we'd complicated our lives in the United States. I was beginning to see that life should be balanced, rich, and rewarding and that we should honor those things above all.

❂–❂–❂

After completing two years at St. George's, I was eligible to take a test from the Educational Commission for Foreign Medical Graduates that would certify me as qualified to continue my studies in a U.S. medical school. I was lucky enough to have a shot at transferring to UCLA for my third year of medical school and did well on the test. When I took part 1 of the board exam—the equivalent test given to U.S. medical students—I passed it on the first try, even though many of my soon-to-be classmates at UCLA had to retake it. Before, I was the outcast who wasn't good enough for U.S. medical school, but now I was passing tests my formerly superior peers had to take twice. The irony wasn't lost on me.

As I started at UCLA, I was excited but terrified. Part of me felt vindicated because I had done so well on the board, while the other part felt as though I were sneaking in through the back door. After all, if I were good enough, I would have gotten into a U.S. medical school right away, wouldn't I? Suddenly, I was in a humongous complex whose maze-like hallways and multiple buildings froze me solid. It was like being dropped off in the middle of New York City for the first time and being told "We have a meeting on the forty-seventh floor of the Chrysler building in twenty minutes; see you there." I was actually stopping patients—as they pushed their IV poles—to ask for directions to a particular building or whether they knew who a certain doctor was. The mixture of fear, excitement, anxiety, and growing self-esteem was overwhelming.

After a while, I saw that UCLA was like any other major teaching hospital—clean, brightly lit, and full of white coats. Little packs of medical students, interns, and residents scurried about doing rounds together, and there was a primary focus on technology.

Technology is fantastic, of course, but with it, the one-on-one aspect of healing the patient can fall by the wayside. In my first year at UCLA, I came across a guy whose lungs sounded terrible—a fine, cracking sound, like a bit of hair slid back and forth through the fingers. The chief resident came in while I was with the patient, and I explained the condition I thought he had using all the big medical words. He had cardiomyopathy with resultant congestive heart failure, and his lung had fluid in the bases. When I finished with my explanation, the resident turned to walk out of the room. "Aren't you going to listen to his lungs?" I asked.

"Yeah, we're going to listen to his lungs," he replied in a tone that made it clear he wouldn't be listening to anyone's lungs. "Let's go down to x-ray."

This became the prime example of an attitude I saw in many doctors. Very few seemed to relish the idea of touching or connecting with the patient. But imagine the healing power in showing some compassion. Imagine how different that scene would have been had the doctor acknowledged the lung sounds and the fact that the patient wasn't feeling well and was probably somewhat frightened. Imagine if we had assured him we were going to look at his x-ray to understand better how to help him. Instead, we filed out of the room without even talking about it. UCLA had high-tech down, but it was far from high-touch.

That year, I received an invitation to go to a professor's house for dinner— a guy named Norman Cousins. I'd never heard of him, but before the dinner, I used my little Macintosh to look him up on the early Internet. It turned out that Cousins wasn't a physician but the chair of the office of psychoneuro-immunology within the department of medicine at UCLA. (I discovered that *psychoneuroimmunology* was the technical term that described the holistic view of medicine I'd explored in acupuncture school and with the bush doctors of Grenada. *Psycho* refers to psychology, *neuro* to the nervous system, and *immuno* to the immune system—so the term describes the interface between a person's thoughts, nervous system, and immune system.) I also saw that Cousins had been editor-in-chief of the *Saturday Review of Literature* and written a book called *Anatomy of an Illness*.

Twenty other students were gathered at his house when I arrived, and Norman and his wife were busy preparing the food. I learned that over the first few months, he was inviting all of the third-year class for dinner. As we ate that evening, we discussed what it meant to be a doctor, what the purpose of a physician was. Norman stated that the purpose of a doctor was "to preserve life."

"There's an ICU on every floor of the center for health sciences, all of which are capable of keeping people alive," I said. "There's got to be more to it than that."

Another guy—a total braniac, though I can't remember his name—agreed with me. "Disease is life," he argued, rattling off a list of diseases that none of us had ever heard of.

*Yeah, that's sort of what I meant*, I thought, thankful to have this fellow student on my side of the debate. In my view, the role of a doctor was to heal, but healing didn't always mean prolonging life, because that was not always possible.

We discussed the topic quite a bit more, but in the end, Norman walked over to me and said, "You know, I think you and I are saying the same thing."

He was right—we *were* saying the same thing; we were just using different language. I was speaking as a physician, he as a non-physician.

Over the next two years, I made a point of attending all of Norman's seminars, and I hung around the psychoneuroimmunology office often. I spent my limited spare time helping with anything that needed to be done, all the way down to sneaking into the surgery office to make copies of fliers for the next department event.

In psychoneuroimmunology, I felt I'd come full circle. I'd found a scientific home for the experiences I'd been trying to collate into Western reductionist thinking. There I was—someone who'd repeated the third grade, gotten special education through high school, struggled with dyslexia, gone to acupuncture school, stuck needles in people to open up "energy channels," and studied with the shamanistic bush doctors of Grenada—at UCLA, feeling that all of these experiences had given me a unique perspective that I was eager to put to use.

●-●-●

During my time at UCLA, I had a pivotal experience that showed me how important it was to not just understand the connectedness of systems in the human body but to also be fully present with each of my patients. It was an experience that made me feel ashamed for years, yet it was crucial to my future philosophy of healing.

At the beginning of the AIDS crisis, none of us really knew what was going on. One day, at the start of the epidemic, I was in the hospital room of a young man who was homosexual and twenty-something—about my age—suffering from a horrific wasting disease. Despite having AIDS, he appeared fit. He had short, dark hair and a confident but guarded manner. My guess was that growing up gay had hardened him in a way. I was new on the wards at the time, and right after I met him, he asked me a simple question: "What's going to happen to me?"

I was not equipped with the tools to answer him. I held his gaze for a moment, shrugged, said some meaningless words, and walked out of the room.

Thinking about that moment chokes me up to this day. I realized my failure as I crossed the threshold, but I couldn't turn back. I felt like a complete and total fraud. I didn't have to know anything: all I had to do was be present and sit with the patient. Talk to him. Listen. But I had failed at that simple task.

The next day, after I had an evening to collect myself and think it through,

I went back into the patient's room. I sat down and said that I realized I had not really answered him the day before and that it was because I hadn't considered the question before entering his room. I was taken off guard and didn't know what to do, I explained. I apologized and asked if he would like to talk. He was silent. His look—half uncomprehending, half angry—still haunts me. As I left the room, I said, "I realize that I failed you yesterday, and I am sorry." He gave no reply.

I decided at that moment that I would treat every patient as if he or she were a loved one of mine around the same age. Is this my brother? My grandpa? Is this my dad? My mom? My sister? (And more recently, is this my grandchild?) I committed to focusing on that relationship in terms of how I communicated with and cared for that person. Physicians are trained to not get emotionally involved, but I say that if you're not emotionally involved, you're a pretty crummy doctor.

●-●-●

After I finished up at UCLA, I moved to Merced, California, to do my residency. Merced is like any small town in America. It's an agricultural community filled with bowlegged guys walking around in boots and cowboy hats and big old belt buckles. But there's also a large population of Hmong refugees from the highland areas of Laos and Vietnam. Soon after I arrived there, I walked into the clinic to find a female nurse trying to take the blood pressure of a Buddhist monk, who was dressed in the full red robe and yellow scarf. She wasn't having much luck. The monk backed away from her every time she tried to put the cuff on him—according to his religion, he wasn't supposed to have contact with women. The nurse wasn't getting it, though, and she had a look on her face like, *Why won't this moron stand still?* It was another one of those moments—like my arrival in Grenada—where I looked at the scene before me, smiled, and thought, *I am home.*

During my three years of residency, I saw a lot of this intersection between traditional cultural healing and modern Western medicine. Some doctors were considering turning several Hmong parents in to Child Protective Services when they found long, streaky bruises on the children's backs, but it wasn't abuse; it was a traditional practice called "coining," in which a person has a silver coin rubbed on his body to aid in healing.

Another time, I was treating a Hmong man for high blood pressure when he exploded at me. He didn't speak English, and I had no idea what was going on. I asked his son to translate for me, but the boy was crying inconsolably. Every time his dad let out a burst of language, the boy cried harder. Eventually, I coaxed it out of him: the father was shouting that I wasn't God, that I couldn't tell him whether he was going to get better or worse. His blood pressure medication was decreasing his risk of stroke or heart attack, but the twelve-year-old son had translated it as, "You've got to take your medicine, Dad, or you're going to die." Because he came from a culture where you stop taking medicine when you're no longer sick, the father didn't understand and probably felt manipulated and lied to. That made sense to me, and it gave me a path from which to work. Sadly, most physicians don't take the time to explore the cause of patients' noncompliance—they had the attitude that many of us are trained to have: "Hey, buddy, my way or the highway."

That isn't to say I was immune from the my-way-or-the-highway attitude. When I started out, I could be an arrogant jerk. Part of me still met patients and thought, *I went to medical school, I'm smart, I know what to do, and if you don't do it . . . what's wrong with you?* I still wasn't looking at the totality of my patients' life experiences and how their past had brought them to the moment they were in. I still wasn't reaching out and understanding what factors in their lives caused them to behave in the ways they were behaving. I was still young. Even though I was doing my best to be present, I hadn't yet grasped the fact that some people had vastly different life experiences from mine—that of a white male from a middle-class family.

During my residency, I was once asked to watch a videotape of me in an appointment with a patient. I was stunned to see that I had my back to the patient throughout most of the meeting. At the time, I was completely engaged in the conversation. I was asking questions, trying to get it all down on paper, but I wasn't even *looking* at this person. I was dumbfounded. I hadn't forgotten the promise I'd made to myself after my interaction with the young man with AIDS. I was present, but I wasn't *showing* that I was present—that I was involved and that I cared—so what difference did it make to the patient?

The behavioral scientist with whom I reviewed the tape didn't seem as distressed as I was—he actually chuckled about it.

"What are you laughing at?" I asked. "This is horrible!"

"Actually, you're doing better than most of them," he replied. "At least you're not interrupting."

He explained that most patients are interrupted within fifteen seconds of beginning to tell their story to a doctor. The fact is that the doctor already knows what he's going to do by the time he sees the nurse's note, and he has another appointment in the next room. So it's, "Yeah, yeah. Here's your prescription. I gotta go." That's the model we have created.

●-●-●

After I finished my residency in 1990, I went into private practice in Lake Tahoe, California. One day, a patient walked through my door and shifted me toward a field that would come to be known as functional medicine.

For six years, this woman had been suffering with chronic pain and fatigue. She'd been diagnosed with chronic fatigue syndrome, which at that time was a new and controversial diagnosis; most people thought it was some kind of psychiatric problem.

She said to me, "Listen, I've seen this guy—Kirk Hamilton. He's a nutritionally oriented doctor."

All through college, I had read Jonathan Wright's work on nutritional medicine and natural treatment of disease, but I had never heard the term "nutritionally oriented doctor."

"Nutritionally oriented?" I asked. "What does he mean by that, exactly?"

"Well, he uses nutrition instead of drugs whenever he can."

I was intrigued. She gave me his name and phone number and told me he took calls from eight to nine in the morning. I called him at eight the next day, and my first impression was that this man clearly had untreated ADD. He was a ball of fire, talking a mile a minute, and seemed to have all the world's literature on nutrition at his fingertips. I learned that he was actually a physician's assistant, not a physician, and he lived down near Davis. He went to the Davis Medical library every month, where he combed through every magazine to find articles about nutrition and holism. He then wrote a monthly newsletter with a blurb about each article and its conclusions.

Through meeting Kirk and reading his newsletter, I re-plugged into the holistic approach that had defined my early forays into medicine. I started attending seminars held by people like Jonathan Wright, Allen Gaby, and Jeffrey Bland, and reading their respective work.

From the time I first saw that woman, it took about a year for me to become fully immersed in functional medicine. By the end of that year, I wasn't some well-rounded expert in holism, but my practice had become dedicated to this holistic, interconnected idea. To this day, the pieces of that very large puzzle continue to fall into place.

Thanks to the discoveries I made in the early parts of my career, I've come to understand that the purpose of a doctor is definitely more than keeping patients alive. Because we now have technological marvels that are wonderful for getting people through short-term crises, we tend to oversell ourselves as physicians, and everybody starts to think they can be saved by medical advances. But we rarely have those careful, compassionate, thoughtful conversations with patients about the disease process. It's those conversations, however, that make all the difference. Real miracles don't come from being hooked up to a ventilator. They occur when a doctor is able to heal a person's life, even if that doesn't necessarily mean curing the disease. Understanding patients as people, helping them create meaning, and creating a path out of dis-ease back to ease—that's the real miracle-work physicians can do.

And that's where functional medicine comes in.

# THE TIMELINE AND THE MATRIX

Most physicians have been trained to practice "acute care"—in other words, they're focused on diagnosing and treating short-term or urgent conditions. You go to the doctor with appendicitis; you get your appendix removed. You go in with a sinus infection; you get a prescription for an antibiotic. The physician sees a problem and prescribes a specific corresponding treatment, such as a medication or surgery. Once your immediate symptom is treated, that's that.

But as we all know, Americans are suffering from an explosion not of acute conditions but *chronic* disease, from cancer to diabetes to mental illness. The acute-care approach doesn't come close to addressing the complicated nature of these conditions. Functional medicine, on the other hand, takes a deeper, more nuanced look—not at the patient's immediate complaint, but at the patients themselves, their complex backgrounds, lifestyles, and environments. Unlike traditional medicine, the functional approach strives to enhance wellness—and if wellness is optimized, disease cannot flourish. I'm convinced it's what all physicians will be practicing fifty years from now—or sooner.

Before they even arrive for their first visit to my practice, our patients are asked to fill out a comprehensive online questionnaire. All the questions require a yes or a no answer—there are no maybes. If you say no, you move on, but if you give the computer a yes, you're prompted to answer a new set of questions about your symptoms and medical history. The goal of the questionnaire is to find when wellness started to diminish, not the time when illness started (generally, there is a big gap between the two). Some patients complain about how long it takes to answer all the questions, but it's crucial that I have a full portrait of what they're experiencing. After all, I'm not just trying to mask a symptom with medication. I'm going to look for patterns and connections. It takes a little effort on the patient's part, but that's why I call what I do "audience participation medicine." It's as if you've come to a theater where the actors expect you to be part of the play.

This approach isn't something patients are used to, as today's traditional physician is far too busy to delve into the causes of a complex condition in a person. He's not trained in the proper methodology or equipped with the necessary tools to treat long-lasting conditions that may be bound up with several simultaneous conditions. He doesn't have the time to delve into the patient's genetic makeup, environment, and exposure to different toxins, or the aspects of the patient's lifestyle that are likely contributing to the condition. Though the physician can match disease to drug, he's not trained to address the root of the problem or prescribe nutritional or exercise strategies—treatments that may, in some cases, be as effective or more so than drugs. Worse yet, his recommendations may be woefully out of date: there is a huge lag between medical research and integration into medical access—sometimes as long as fifty years. And the gap is particularly wide in the treatment of persistent, complex, chronic diseases.

A patient who makes an appointment with a functional medicine doctor—usually after several exhausting acute-care visits—finds a wholly different style of addressing the problem at hand. The practitioner is conversant in the latest research. He asks abundant questions and listens closely to the answers. He's focused on the body as an integrated system, not as a collection of independent organs. He treats disease not as an anomalous quirk but as the body's natural effort to normalize physiology in the face of a mismatched genetic makeup and environment. But let's take a step back.

In my office, the very first difference patients notice is the atmosphere. We ditched the sterile, unwelcoming whites and grays of the traditional doctor's office in favor of a large, open reception area painted in vibrant greens and yellows. Plants populate the corners of the room, and large photos of tulips hang on the walls. We stock a wide selection of vitamins and nutritional supplements—used to control inflammation, high cholesterol, high blood sugar, and many other conditions—on a large shelf, but there are no drug advertisements. We want people to be struck by the healing energy of the room. We want it to be a far cry from how they feel when they step into to the drab atmosphere that plagues most waiting rooms.

On top of that, we make sure our staff members treat patients with true empathy and leave their own problems at the door. Too often, distressed patients are subjected to grousing and gossiping at the front desk or the nurses' station, which only increases the patients' anxiety and frustration. For that reason, we insist that our employees focus only on the patient once they cross the threshold. If one of us is having a bad day, we take a deep breath, center ourselves, and do our best to move forward with a healing attitude. If that's not possible, we go home.

It may seem extreme, but that's what we're here for—to help the patient heal. Because we practice functional medicine, we give patient-centered care. We don't want to just rid people of disease. We want them to regain vitality and true health. And to do that, we have to get to know them quite deeply. That all starts in the first appointment, where functional medicine doctors deploy two key tools: the timeline and the matrix.

●-●-●

When I first met Jared, he was thirty-two years old and sickly looking, with dark circles collecting shadows beneath his eyes. At five eleven and one hundred and seventy-five pounds, he was perhaps a bit underweight for the average American, though the weight itself was healthy. He seemed preoccupied and distant; eye contact was infrequent.

"So, what brings you here today?" I asked.

"Well," he said, gaze fixed on the floor, "I have asthma. I've had it for about five years. I've tried several approaches, but nothing's really helped."

This one- to two-sentence answer, followed by silence, is something I see often, and it's a direct effect of the traditional approach to medicine. Patients have been trained to encapsulate their medical history and describe their symptoms briefly for an overbooked doctor, who then prescribes something and is on his way. But those two sentences tell me almost nothing. To learn about the patient's condition, you have to dig deeper.

The next question I asked is one that all functional medicine doctors use in the first visit: "When was the last time you felt truly well?"

"Hmm." Jared chewed his lip. "About five years ago is when the asthma really started giving me big problems."

"So, before five years ago, you were doing pretty well?"

"Actually, I guess not," said Jared. "I've had irritable bowel syndrome since I was a kid."

"So, taking the IBS into account, when was the last time you felt truly well?"

Jared thought for a moment before meeting my eyes. "If you're being *that* detailed," he said, "probably not since the sixth grade."

Now I had the answer to what I call the "not well since" question. I use that as the jumping-off point. "Tell me about fifth grade," I said.

Jared shook his head, almost laughing. "That was almost two decades ago," he said. "I don't know. It was fine."

He was obviously reluctant—not because he was hiding anything but because he felt as though he would be wasting my time with his childhood memories. I smiled back at him. "Humor me."

"Well," he said, eyebrows knitting together, "I could do whatever I wanted, eat whatever I wanted. I was an active kid. It wasn't until sixth grade, about halfway through the year, that I got sick."

I now had the starting point for Jared's timeline (see figure 1). I took out a blank sheet of paper and snapped it to my clipboard. The timeline sheet shows a long line labeled "Triggers or Triggering Events," with a short section at the far left marked "Antecedents." The Antecedents section is for genetic factors and family history; it would hold the predispositions with which Jared was born. The beginning of the long Triggers section represented Jared's life and would hold the occurrences that triggered his various conditions. I added a point in the childhood area near approximately sixth grade and wrote "IBS."

The conversation moved forward as I teased more information out of Jared. He was actually a physician himself, though in Physician Land, a thirty-two-year-old is barely out of school. When he was diagnosed with adult-onset asthma five years earlier, he'd been given several inhalers, which somewhat improved his condition. A year later, he got a stool test—he was still living with IBS—and was found to have the parasite *Blastocystis hominis* and an overgrowth of yeast. He was treated with an antifungal and Metronidazole to kill off the *Blastocystis*, and after that, he noticed significant improvement in his IBS symptoms. All those events became data points—triggers—on the timeline I was filling out.

Unfortunately, Jared's reprieve from IBS was short-lived. A year later, his symptoms slowly returned, worsening until they reached a low point about six

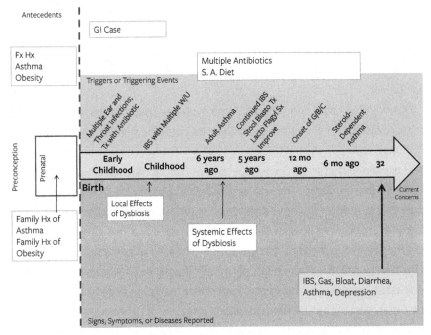

Figure 1

months before he came to see me. But Jared came to me not to address his IBS but to address his asthma—he'd lived with the IBS since sixth grade and had come to view the condition as normal. Jared also told me that he'd been suffering from recurrent depression. It was becoming apparent to me that his conditions—primarily the asthma, IBS, and depression—were probably linked.

I now had the basics down on the timeline, but Jared's resistance to sharing details with me wasn't going away. He seemed to want to give me a neat little summary of his condition, get a prescription, and leave, even though I knew he'd come to me because he'd heard I was different. I sensed he didn't quite think I was legit. I was asking him a ton of questions, but he'd give me one little tidbit of information and then clam up. Most patients have the opposite reaction—they're delighted to find that I'm actually hearing their story and asking questions. They say things like "Wow! You're the first doctor who's really listened to me. I always thought these things were connected, but nobody took me seriously!" But Jared, as a physician himself, was initially resistant to the functional medicine approach.

After getting a particularly abbreviated answer, I stopped. "Jared," I said, "I'm trying to get the big picture of what's going on with you. All this stuff is potentially highly interrelated. We've got forty-five minutes, not five. I want more than a snapshot. Asthma is an inflammatory disease—don't you think your gut is inflamed when you're having an attack of IBS?"

Jared's eyes flicked to the corner where wall met ceiling. "Yeah," he said. "Probably."

"Definitely," I said. "And there's some evidence that depression is an inflammatory disease of the brain, so I think that could be related, too."

"Okay . . ."

I explained that from the perspective of functional medicine, medical specialties were outdated. The way we divide and classify these specialties, each addressing a different type of disease, is an antiquated holdover from the ancient Greeks. We now know that most diseases are "multi-system," meaning they're not isolated to a single specialized area of conventional medicine. This silo approach is at the heart of modern medicine's failure to treat chronic disease. I explained to Jared that functional medicine organizes disease not by organ system but by fundamental physiological process—such as inflammation, biotransformation, communication, and so on. This is a better fit for the reality of disease: heart disease, gastrointestinal (GI) disease, and skin disease may all share a similar foundational cause, and three different people's heart disease may have three different causes.

My explanation hit home. Jared was finally ready to talk more. It turned out he'd had several ear infections as a child, as well as a family history of chronic sinusitis and asthma. There was also a history of obesity on his mother's side of the family. All this pointed to Jared having a strong genetic predisposition to inflammatory conditions.

We also delved into his lifestyle. Jared told me he was living on carbs and caffeine, a trend that had started in childhood. As an adult, he often picked up fast food at the drive-through, rarely exercised, never ate fish, and popped Tums frequently. He also told me he took aspirin several times a week for joint and muscle pain. At that point, it wasn't lost on either of us that aspirin is anti-inflammatory.

I continued pushing Jared for details, asking things like "Did I get this right?" and "Do I understand that?" He doled out specifics reluctantly, but each time I got a new piece of information, I entered it into the timeline.

During the process, Jared also started opening up about what it was like to live with some of these conditions. "It's not fun to go to a buddy's house for a sleepover as a kid and worry the whole time about having an accident," he said, explaining how the condition had made him feel marginalized, different from everyone else. It extended to his adult life, too—it was embarrassing to excuse himself to use the restroom and be gone for thirty minutes. Since the worsening of his asthma and IBS about six months before his visit with me, Jared had been on a strict diet, which made the social awkwardness even worse. He couldn't even have lunch with colleagues—he'd have to tell them that, no thanks, he couldn't go because he brought his own rice and water, the only foods he thought would improve his stomach condition.

Jared was on what I call the "fearful diet"—a diet in which you desperately try to figure out what's causing your symptoms and are fearful that any food you eat may cause a flare-up. You know how it goes: "Well, last time I ate soy, my stomach was fine, but this time I got sick. I probably shouldn't eat soy." It's like getting the flu after eating spaghetti and swearing off spaghetti for two years.

By this point, I'd fleshed out Jared's timeline significantly. All of his various ailments were noted linearly across the page, allowing us to see a picture of his whole medical history at a glance. Soon, we made our first breakthrough.

Jared, like most patients and physicians—and he was both—had been trained to see everything in isolation. Though he'd come in because of his asthma, he hadn't realized that it was inextricably linked to the IBS. As we looked at the timeline, I asked how his asthma had been in the year-long reprieve he'd had from IBS following the treatment of the *Blastocystis* parasite in his gut.

"You know what?" Jared mused. "It was entirely gone that year."

There it was. Our first "aha" moment. The timeline had helped Jared make an important connection. "Did you ever think about getting retested for those parasites?" I asked.

"No . . . it never occurred to me," said Jared. Then, almost instantly, he turned defensive: "But I'm not entirely convinced it's possible that that's the cause."

It was going to take a little work to show him that the connection was real, but I knew he'd seen the connection between his asthma and his bowel problems for the first time. Insights like this one are why the timeline is so useful. So often, a patient will come in and say something like "I know Lipitor is what caused all my problems!" I'll then ask them when the problem started, and they'll say it was January 4, 2001. But when I ask when they started Lipitor, they'll say it was about the middle of 2003. When the patient sees the timeline, they see that this connection doesn't make sense, but that's just how the brain works; it doesn't always view things rationally. *I read this is a side effect of Lipitor,* your brain tells you, *so Lipitor must be the problem.* No other facts are relevant until you see them on paper.

●-●-●

The process I went through with Jared is much like what functional medicine doctors do with every patient. I'm not so much interested in what's bothering you right now as I am in who you are, what your history is, and what your environment and lifestyle are like. I'm interested in how you got to your current state of health because that will help us plot a path back to real health.

Once I have a sense of that, it's time for the physical exam. This part of the visit is generally not long and drawn out, since my patients have seen multiple doctors and had many exams already, of which I have the records. However, I do a nutritionally centered physical exam and examine portions of the body that I feel are relevant based on the initial discussion. In Jared's case, I looked at his nose and found that the nasal mucus membrane was boggy, swollen, and red. Inside his mouth, his pharynx—the part of the throat right below the mouth and nose—was inflamed and red. I also noticed that his skin was dry and that he had a cobblestone texture on the back of his arms and white spots on his fingernails. I then listened to five or six places on his chest, as I'd been taught by my mentors in Grenada. Jared's heart rate and everything else I found in the remainder of the physical exam was normal.

The next step was filling out Jared's matrix. I fill out a matrix (see figure 2) for each of my patients; it's a helpful way for me to encapsulate the person's condition in a holistic way. In the center of the circle is a space for listing antecedents (in Jared's case, antibiotics and a propensity for inflammation) as well as triggers, of which Jared had an abundance, including the *Blastocystis hominis* parasite, the recurrent depression, and the aspirin and Tums he used to medicate his symptoms. There, I also listed the mediators—the intermediary factors that perpetuate the illness.

Eight points surrounded the circle at the center of the matrix, each sector representing a piece of Jared's health. Using the timeline, I filled in the relevant sectors of the matrix; for Jared, my marks were mainly in the categories of

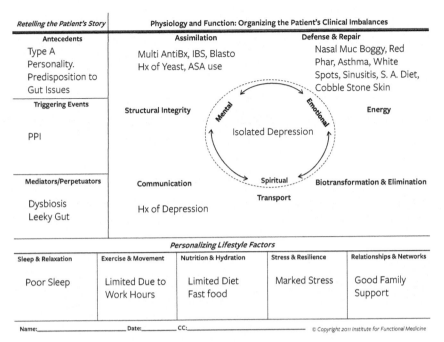

| Retelling the Patient's Story | Physiology and Function: Organizing the Patient's Clinical Imbalances | | |
|---|---|---|---|
| **Antecedents** | **Assimilation** | | **Defense & Repair** |
| Type A Personality. Predisposition to Gut Issues | Multi AntiBx, IBS, Blasto Hx of Yeast, ASA use | | Nasal Muc Boggy, Red Phar, Asthma, White Spots, Sinusitis, S. A. Diet, Cobble Stone Skin |
| **Triggering Events** | Structural Integrity | *Mental* Isolated Depression *Emotional* | Energy |
| PPI | | | |
| **Mediators/Perpetuators** | Communication | Spiritual Transport | Biotransformation & Elimination |
| Dysbiosis Leeky Gut | Hx of Depression | | |

| *Personalizing Lifestyle Factors* | | | | |
|---|---|---|---|---|
| Sleep & Relaxation | Exercise & Movement | Nutrition & Hydration | Stress & Resilience | Relationships & Networks |
| Poor Sleep | Limited Due to Work Hours | Limited Diet Fast food | Marked Stress | Good Family Support |

Name:_____ Date:_____ CC:_____    © Copyright 2011 Institute for Functional Medicine

Figure 2

- **Assimilation** (Digestion, Absorption, and Barrier Integrity): the parasite, his IBS, his history of intestinal yeast, the antibiotics he'd been treated with, and the Tums he ate so often;

- **Defense and Repair** (Inflammatory Processes): his asthma, his depression, the family history of obesity and sinusitis, the texture of his skin, the swollen nasal membrane, the inflamed pharynx, the white spots on his fingernails, his aspirin usage, his poor diet, and the food sensitivity I suspected; and

- **Mental, Emotional, and Spiritual**: Jared's depression and slow social life.

Finally, I duplicated "depression" in the hormone and neurotransmitter regulation (Communication) section of the matrix.

Jared and I conversed as I filled out his matrix, and when I was done, I shared some of my speculations with him. I explained that because he'd been treated with antibiotics as a kid, his gut flora may have been altered, which may have led to his IBS. I also explained that, based on his family history, I thought he was predisposed to atopic disease—meaning he had a tendency to develop allergic reactions (including asthma). I told him that his mediators—factors that perpetuate his conditions—were the aspirin, his depression, and his poor diet.

Jared nodded, chewing his cheek, and said no when I asked if he had any questions.

Now I brought out a new blank matrix and filled it out not with his symptoms but with the underlying conditions I suspected had caused them. Under Digestion, Absorption, and Barrier Integrity, I explained that I thought he had a condition called dysbiosis, which was probably causing leaky gut. I told him that leaky gut can cause abnormal interactions between the immune system and the gut content.

"Think of it like this," I said. "Put your hands in front of your eyes with the fingers close together."

I demonstrated. Jared looked at me skeptically but raised his hands, blocking me from his line of sight.

"Now, your eyes are your immune system looking into your gut—it can't see much. The bacteria in your gut is camouflaged as you. It looks to your immune system as if it belongs. That's a healthy gut. Now open your fingers."

Jared's dark eyes peeked at me through the gaps between his fingers.

"Now that the 'camouflaged' stuff is easily seen, your immune system may start to make antibodies against it. The problem is because it looks like you, your immune system may make antibodies that react to the real you as well as the stuff that doesn't belong. That's autoimmunity, which brings us to the next section."

Under the Defense and Repair sector of the second matrix, I wrote that he likely had food sensitivities and a zinc deficiency (one known sign of zinc deficiency is white spots on the fingernails). Next, we moved up to the Defense and Repair sector, where I noted that in addition to a likely predisposition to inflammation, he probably wasn't getting enough fatty acids (since he never ate fish) or zinc.

Thanks to the matrix, we now had a basic picture of how all of Jared's problems might interrelate. For the first time, he was seeing how deeply connected his asthma and IBS were—they'd likely both been kicked off by the childhood antibiotics and worsened by *Blastocystis hominis* and food sensitivities. Jared had found the matrix enlightening, but like all patients, he was eager to get to the next question—how do we start reversing this mess?

To find the answer, I took Jared for a third and final spin around his matrix.

This time, at each sector, I told him what we might investigate. I told him we could run tests for gut permeability, gut digestive function, and food sensitivity, and do a fatty acid analysis and test for the presence of parasites. It was a lot of testing, and Jared looked a bit overwhelmed when I was finished outlining the complete plan.

"Listen," I told him, "don't worry—we don't have to do this all at once. My hunch is that this all hinges on the parasites. Let's start there. If that doesn't get you better, we'll move on to the rest of it."

Now that we had a path forward, it was time for the next step in the visit. It was time for me to tell Jared his story.

# Chapter 3

# THE STORY

Every one of my patients has a story, complete with a setting, plot, key characters, and important themes. As a physician, I'm interested in how the events in the patient's story got him where he is today—namely, suffering from disease and in my office, desperate for help. The patient has lived that story, but it's usually difficult for him to step back and spot the connections within it; yet those connections are often the beginning of a holistic treatment plan for the problems—physical, spiritual, and emotional—that brought the patient to me in the first place.

Once I've completed a patient's timeline and matrix, I sit down and retell his story, from beginning to present. We move from when he last felt good to the current state of feeling bad, and we then lay out a new path back to feeling good. I've found that using the story as the centerpiece of my relationship with the patient has benefits beyond promoting understanding; often, it is the key to reigniting the patient's hope and helping him stick to a treatment plan.

## JARED'S STORY

I'd learned a lot about Jared's story as we built his timeline and matrix, and once we were done, it was time for me to present it to him.

"Okay, Jared," I said. "I think I have a pretty good picture of what's happening here, and now I want to work through it with you. Sound okay?"

"Yeah," said Jared. He'd opened up slightly since the beginning of his visit, and I could tell by his forward lean that he was engaged, but I still sensed his hesitation. He was a doctor himself, after all, and he still wasn't completely on board with my methods.

"It won't be just me telling you a story, though," I said. "It's actually going to be more of a conversation. So if I say something that doesn't seem quite right, I want you to chime in and let's talk about that piece." I wanted Jared to listen intently, to have ownership of the story.

Jared agreed, and I began.

"As a physician, I'm sure you have heard of 'high-reliability organizations,' right?"

Jared nodded. Physicians know that every organization in healthcare strives to be high reliability—in other words, an organization that has succeeded in avoiding accidents and major disasters despite operating in an environment where such occurrences are common.

"One of the most extreme environments, in terms of safety, is an aircraft carrier," I continued. "Yet, aircraft carriers have had an unparalleled safety record because of the integrated systems they've put into place to maintain safety. They've become high-reliability organizations. For a catastrophe to occur, multiple mistakes—chains of mistakes—have to occur. The human body is very similar: each step in its chemical and biological processes serves as a double-check to ensure that previous mistakes have not been made. So, it's a high-reliability system with multiple checks and balances, and in order for something to go wrong, multiple mistakes must have been made, with the checks and balances failing as well. In your case, before you contracted IBS or asthma, several things had gone awry, all of which caused problems later. It's not unlike a line of dominos. Once the process starts, the dominos fall until they reach the end. Our job is to understand that path—to trace our way back to that first fallen domino. That will help us plot a course back to wellness."

"Okay," said Jared. He was watching me intensely, and I got a glimpse of the kind of student he'd been in medical school: cynical but engaged. I could tell he was curious about what I had to say next.

"You came to me because of your asthma, but it looks to me like there's a longer chain of events that brought us to this meeting. It really starts before your birth, with both genetic and epigenetic issues." Epigenetics, as I knew Jared understood, is the study of heritable changes in gene expression caused by mechanisms other than changes in the underlying DNA sequence—in other words, the idea that our parents' lifestyle decisions can affect our health outside the perinatal phase. I could see him tense at the E-word, but he didn't say anything. To most traditional physicians, talking about epigenetics is tantamount to bringing up Lamarckism—the still-controversial idea that an organism can pass on to its offspring traits it developed within its lifetime.

"In your case, you have a family history of asthma and obesity. More and more evidence suggests that obesity is an inflammatory disease. The epigenetic consequence of this family history is likely a pro-inflammatory environment in your body. Asthma, as you know, is also an inflammatory disease, and this is a second source of a predisposition to inflammation in your body. Then you told me you'd had multiple recurrent ear infections as a child, which were treated with antibiotics. While these antibiotics cured your ear infections, they also disrupted your gut microflora, and the development of your immune system depends on healthy gut microflora.

"In addition, disordered microflora—or 'dysbiosis'—can result in hyperpermeability of the gut, called 'leaky gut.' This leaky gut can result in abnormal interactions between the stuff that normally lives in your intestines and your immune system. This is another inflammatory condition, and it can lead to many environmental sensitivities.

"Imagine a hunter out in the woods dressed in camouflage. If the hunter is motionless and kneeling by a bush that matches the spots on his camo, he's hard to see. However, the same hunter wearing the same camouflage and standing in the middle of a parking lot would be easy to spot because he's out of place. In much the same way, the microorganisms that live in our gut are camouflaged—they have spots on them that make them look very much like us. When you have leaky gut, the bugs inside you are like the hunter standing in the parking lot: easily visible to your immune system. Unfortunately, because the bugs were camouflaged to look like you, some of the antibodies you make inadvertently attack you. This process is known as 'molecular mimicry,' and it's likely the origin of many autoimmune diseases. It also results in even more inflammation, and food sensitivities caused by leaky gut further escalate the inflammatory process.

"The immune system within the gut is used to seeing fully digested food," I continued. "In the presence of leaky gut, the immune system comes in contact with partially digested food, and these larger molecules are not recognized as normal healthy food but as possible invaders. In an effort to protect itself from these partially digested foods, the body mounts a defensive reaction and in so doing creates yet more inflammation."

Jared leaned back in his chair and folded his lanky arms across his chest. "But nobody really knows why autoimmunity happens. I mean, I'm an internist, and—not to be disrespectful—I've never heard anything remotely similar to this."

"Look," I said, "not to be disrespectful either, but clinicians don't look into this stuff enough. It's not in our literature; it's in the more basic science literature. Before you leave, I'm going to print up a few papers—peer-reviewed papers, by the way—that discuss this. Molecular mimicry is one of several mechanisms by which we think autoimmunity happens, but I'm not just pulling this out of thin air. It's emerging science, and I believe it's likely that this process originally led to your irritable bowel syndrome. You then limped along with IBS for many years, and at some point, you contracted *Blastocystis*, normally a fairly benign parasite. But in the face of your pro-inflammatory predisposition and leaky gut, it became more pathogenic. This increasing inflammatory burden eventually manifested itself as asthma, bringing you here today."

Jared scoffed audibly. "Come on! I mean, I followed this for a while, but that's ridiculous."

I was taken aback momentarily. Usually the response I get is "I had no idea" or "Holy cow, I never thought of that."

Then I remembered that I was dealing with a doubting Thomas, which was to be expected given Jared's background in traditional medicine. Some of what I was saying, especially about the connection between gut flora and asthma, would have been totally new to him. Often, the physician's mentality is "I'm smart, I went to medical school. If I haven't heard of it, it must be bullshit." (That's why most of them write off chiropractors and naturopaths. Those fields aren't part of their training, so it's got to be wrong, right?) Nevertheless, I knew he was interested and didn't think I was entirely a fraud. Why else would he be in my office?

Whatever the case, I had to show Jared I was serious and that I knew the literature, so I turned again to peer-reviewed medical journals. I took him back through a chain of evidence, demonstrating how others had shown that, yes, *Blastocystis*—the parasite he had—does, in fact, have variable pathogenicity and can affect gut permeability; that gut permeability has been linked to asthma; and that probiotics have been shown to decrease gut permeability. My printer hummed as it spat out fresh pages for Jared to take home and read.

"The root of all this, I think, is the dysbiosis, the imbalance of the bacteria in your gut," I said. "Either the *Blastocystis* or some other parasite has regrown and is causing the inflammation that's the root of the IBS and the asthma. I want to do a parasite test on your stool and then some other basic interventions to get your inflammation under control. I think we should get you on a probiotic—an immunoglobulin—and also cut out a bunch of different foods in an elimination diet."

Jared's face fell at the last two words. Getting him past the idea that I was a quack was one obstacle, but as we moved toward the topic of changing his diet, I wondered if we'd hit an even bigger challenge. Though Jared was a doctor, the food he ate was uniformly atrocious, and the elimination diet (technically called an oligoantigenic diet) would knock out tons of commonly eaten foods, precisely because the commonly eaten ones also happen to be the ones we get sensitized to most frequently. Most of Jared's former diet—much of which was procured from a drive through—would be wiped out.

"Oh god," said Jared when I gave him a handout summarizing the foods he could and couldn't have and outlining suggested recipes and menus.

"Bear with me here," I said. "We'll go through this together." We started on the forbidden foods side. "Okay," I began, "let's just run through the things you need to stay away from. No corn or corn products. No eggs. No dairy products—that includes milk, cheese, ice cream, yogurt, frozen yogurt. No beef, pork, veal. No cold cuts, canned meats, hot dogs, frankfurters. No peanuts or peanut products, no soybeans or soybean products."

Patients typically start to fidget during this part, and I know exactly what's going through their heads: What the hell can I eat? (One patient said to me, "I know why they call it a comprehensive elimination diet—because it comprehensively eliminates everything I like to eat!") I was going on and on, and I saw the familiar fatigue on Jared's face.

"I know what you're thinking," I said, trying to beat him to the punch. "What's left?"

Jared laughed. "You got it."

"Well, turn that page over and let's see. This is your shopping list. You can have as many of these foods as you like. So here are fruits. You can have any of these, from apples all the way down to watermelon. And here are the vegetables, artichokes to zucchini. In the other column, there are grain substitutes; they're all gluten-free. So you can have amaranth and millet and quinoa and teff and buckwheat."

Jared silently scanned the handout, hardly looking excited about expanding his grain-substitute repertoire.

"For proteins," I continued, "you can have free-range chicken, turkey, or duck. You can have fresh fish caught wild from the ocean—"

"Just the ocean?" Jared interrupted. "What about fresh water fish?"

"Fish caught from the ocean are best studied and have the most anti-inflammatory properties," I said. "Plus, fresh water suffers more from pollution. Here in Minnesota, it's recommended that you eat only one serving of freshwater fish per week if you're not pregnant and one per month if you are because of mercury levels. That's just ridiculous!"

Jared nodded, but I could tell his mind was still on the list of can- and cannot-eats I was giving him. "Okay, you can also have water-packed tuna, lamb, and wild game. I know a lot of these aren't common foods, but that's the point of this whole thing."

As I explained to Jared, it's not that there's anything *wrong* with the foods the elimination diet forbids; the problem is that these are the most commonly eaten foods in our culture and, thus, the foods to which we are most frequently sensitized. Eating foods we're sensitized to results in increased inflammation, which results in more gut leakiness, which in turn results in more sensitivity. It's like a dog chasing its tail. By eliminating all the likely culprits for a few months and then systematically adding them back, one by one, we can figure out what we're sensitized to, stop eating those foods, and reduce inflammation and promote healing of the gut. When the gut begins to heal, the immune system is re-isolated from the gut content, and there are fewer abnormal interactions between the gut content and the immune system, reducing the whole inflammatory process and allowing the lining of the gut to heal.

After explaining all this to Jared, I moved on to describing how he'd start reintroducing foods after three months on the diet—assuming he was feeling good. He'd start by adding back single-ingredient foods (i.e., not pizza) one at a time, every four days. That four-day window allows for any delayed reaction that a given food might cause—sometimes it takes forty-eight hours, and then you want forty-eight hours for any potential reaction to abate before you move on to the next food.

If you add a food and nothing happens, you can safely leave it in your diet. If you're not sure whether you had a reaction (Am I really feeling bad, or is this just a crappy day?), then the food goes back on the list to try again in a week or two. If you try it again and you again have a reaction or semi-reaction, it goes back on the list for another shot in three months. Once it's confirmed you have a reaction, that food is officially out, though not forever—just until your gut is healed.

"I've got to admit—I don't know if I can do this," Jared said, slapping the sheet of paper against his thigh. "I'm really, really busy. I don't know if I could stick to a diet even if I wanted to."

"Well, I can't force you to do it," I said, "but I think it's going to be virtually impossible to solve your problem without dietary change. Following this is going to cut to the heart of a lot of your problems, whether you believe me or not. We need to attack this leaky gut at the source. Imagine it like this. There's an old man walking in the woods, and he comes upon a young man trying to cut down a tree. This young guy is swinging his axe with all of his might and not getting very far. The old man says, 'Gee, son, that must be a hard tree.' The young man replies, 'No, my axe is dull.' 'Why don't you sharpen the axe?' the old man asks. The young man says, 'I don't have time.' Now how silly is that? But you have a dull axe, Jared, and you're going to need to sharpen it, unless you want to waste a lot more time and effort."

Jared emitted a long-suffering sigh before nodding grimly. "Okay. I'll try."

## THE STORY AND ADHERENCE

The elimination diet is quite a haul for most people. Where there's a will, there's a way, but unfortunately, the inverse is true, too: where there is no will, there is often no way. The functional medicine approach, and the axe story in particular, help immensely in my efforts to get patients to stick with a treatment protocol. The story gives meaning and understanding in a practical way. It reignites the patient's curiosity and rekindles hope. When told artfully, the story contains everything the patient needs to move forward, including the will to make hard changes.

Most physicians will tell you they can't get their patients to follow a diet. I always want to say, "Well that's because you hand them a diet sheet and walk out of the room!" I, and most physicians who practice functional medicine, know that to promote adherence to a diet, or any other step we recommend, you have to convince the patient that it's important. It's not enough to know why and how he should shift to healthier behaviors—people have known they shouldn't smoke for decades, but they do because smoking won't kill them today. Education isn't enough. Patients must be inspired by the meaning behind treatment; they must feel hope that the difficult changes will give them a better life. You can't just follow the old routine: see the patient for 18.5 nanoseconds, hand him a prescription, and be on your way. No meaning was created in that interaction. Showing the patient you understand his story by retelling it—and together plotting the path from the darkness and despair of disease to full wellness—can make the difference between adherence and abandonment of the treatment plan.

Embedded in the story I told Jared were clear reasons for making the change. We discussed at length how he'd become sensitive to many of the foods he was eating regularly—even some of the non–fast food items, such as grains and fruit. I reminded Jared about his leaky gut and the immune system's interactions with partially digested foods. I explained that people with leaky gut frequently become sensitive to foods they commonly eat—even if those foods are healthy ones. We also made sure that when Jared left our office, he was equipped to change his story and have a much more positive chapter to share when he came back in five weeks. That's where my lifestyle educator came in.

The lifestyle educator pulled even more details out of Jared's story and helped him develop solutions for how he could change his approach in the coming weeks.

"What do you normally do for dinner?" she asked first, starting with what is usually the largest meal of the day.

"Well, I used to stop at McDonald's on the way back from work," said Jared, "but I know that's terrible. I've gotten a lot better. I still eat out a lot, but it's better stuff. For instance, Applebee's has a good low-calorie takeout menu."

From there, they worked out a better solution: he could stop at the grocery store deli on the way back from work and pick up an elimination-diet friendly dinner there. It was a little less convenient, but Jared agreed it was doable.

Next the lifestyle educator asked, "What about when you get home? Do you have an evening snack?"

Jared's reply revealed another less-than-ideal habit. "Yeah, most nights I eat something sweet."

"Have you heard of Rice Dream ice cream?" she asked, smiling. "It's like ice cream, but it's acceptable on the elimination diet and will help you feel less deprived." Then she proposed another, even better option: a handful of nuts or berries.

Jared nodded and offered a small smile in return. As he saw that he wasn't going to be subsisting on celery sticks and bran for the next five weeks, I could tell we were getting more buy-in. The lifestyle educator moved on: he could replace toast and coffee for breakfast with gluten-free bread and any of a selection of teas allowed on the elimination diet. And if he was in a pinch, he could eat a medical food we gave him, a quick, convenient way to get protein and antioxidants. The medical food we use is a powder that's reconstituted in water or juice, and it's intended for the dietary management of disease that has nutritional needs that a regular diet wouldn't cover. To replace his usual midmorning candy bar, Jared could make sure he brought an apple or some blueberries to work each day. In fact, he could pick up all the fruit he needed for the week when he stopped at the grocery store deli for dinner.

Lunch had a similar solution: rather than buying a sandwich and chips from the vendor who came by the hospital, he could eat a chicken breast or a piece of fish he brought from home. The lifestyle educator encouraged him to cook up a bunch of chicken or fish at the same time—that way he'd have several days' worth prepared. It was going to take more effort than simply switching from Big Macs to McNuggets, but Jared seemed on board and willing to give it a try.

The next subject was exercise. Jared wasn't a regular at the gym, and he wasn't especially active, so we started him off easy and asked him to take a twenty-minute walk every day. No mention of intensity or anything else—just a twenty-minute stroll. "You can do it first thing when you get up; you can do it on your lunch break; you can do it right after work; you can do it in the evening," said the lifestyle educator. "Just make sure you do it." The lifestyle educator also encouraged Jared to find activities that he truly enjoys and do those as a form of exercise. Most people get their best workouts during activities they don't even regard as exercise, whether it's working in the garden, rollerblading with a friend, or going dancing.

Finally, we needed to talk to Jared about taking his probiotics each day. Though you'd think swallowing a pill would be simple, especially in comparison to the dietary shifts we were recommending for Jared, a huge number of patients simply don't take the medications prescribed to them. Yet adherence to the drug therapy is paramount—in fact, studies involving groups on real drugs and groups on a placebo show that the most important factor in improvement isn't whether the drug is real or not but whether the patient adheres to the therapy.

So how could we get Jared to follow the plan and take his probiotics regularly? Again, the answer was "story." I'd explained that probiotics would help his inflamed gut heal by making its lining less permeable, and even if he was still something of skeptic, he understood my explanation as it related to the bigger leaky gut problem I was sure he had. We also encouraged Jared to make taking them a ritual in which he consciously acknowledged the good the pills were doing him each time he swallowed one rather than grousing about the inconvenience. If no one's told you your story, you're likely to just see drug therapy as a hassle and a burden; but when you understand why you're on the drug and how it's improving your health, you approach it with an attitude of gratitude and optimism, not frustration. Think of it this way: If you're holding a few pills in your hand, you can think "I hate taking these pills," or you can think "Thank you for the opportunity to take these medicines that help me feel healthier." Which attitude do you think is most beneficial?

In the end, how much we recommend the patient do between the first and second visit depends on his attitude. Some people are overwhelmed just taking supplements; with them, I'll hold off on the diet till later. The diet pushes some people over the edge, so for them, we'll leave exercise to the second or third visit. But others are ready to climb the mountain right away. Their attitude is, *This is great! Bring it on! I'm totally ready for this!* With them, I'll go for the full-meal deal.

When Jared stepped out of my office with his assignment for the next five weeks and print-outs of several articles on molecular mimicry, he left with an understanding of his story and the knowledge that, if he adhered to the treatment plan, he would likely feel at least 50 percent better next time I saw him. We felt as if we'd done all we could to give him the best chance of success. Part of that was the mechanisms we put in place—for example, the lifestyle educator would be calling him every day for the first week to see how things were going—but the bigger part of it was the story. The one we'd shared with Jared was about a situation he knew well, but we'd added new details (like the *Blastocystis* circumstance that had likely caused his asthma) and shifted his perspective. We'd developed a streamlined narrative that would help Jared move forward and understand his health objectives. The functional medicine approach to telling that story is a world away from the typically impersonal, rushed, and compartmentalized recommendations you'd get from a traditional physician.

And like any good story, the ones I tell my patients involve plenty of metaphor. It's a tool I use to inject even more meaning into the story. Metaphor is powerful. Imagine I said I know two kids in a "Romeo and Juliet" situation. You automatically have an abundance of information and know exactly what I'm talking about. You think of romance, warring families, first love, teenage love, forbidden love, doomed love. I've only said three words, but by invoking a metaphor, I've given you a story that you immediately grasp.

I could say to a patient, "You have idiopathic thrombocytopenic purpura, and we're going to give you prednisone, a glucocorticoid steroid anti-inflammatory medication. The side effects include water retention, hunger, weight gain, and occasionally hallucinations." Lots of doctors do say things like that. But where's the meaning there? How likely is that patient to take the prednisone? A metaphor would give the patient the same information in a much more memorable and persuasive package. Why don't we say something like this instead: "You have idiopathic thrombocytopenic purpura, which means your immune system is really irritated. It's like when a small army is suddenly surrounded by the enemy—it's going to shoot first and ask questions later. Sometimes when the army is overwhelmed, the soldiers accidentally shoot their own guys—it's called friendly fire. That's what's happening in your immune system. It feels overwhelmed right now, so it's shooting at you accidentally. That's called autoimmune disease."

I used metaphor with Jared, especially when I was encouraging him to improve his diet. "If we don't get you off of these foods that are causing inflammation," I told him, "you're going to keep cutting at that tree with your dull axe. We'll never get it under control." It's a simple illustration, but so much more effective than handing off a meal plan and saying good-bye. Every time Jared was tempted to pull in under the Golden Arches, I wanted him to think about his dull axe and how he was working to sharpen it.

## THE STORY AND HOPE

Repeating Jared's story back to him helped build a partnership between him and me, helped him see his history in a new light, and increased the chances that he'd adhere to the plan we set up for him. But the story had another benefit: it gave Jared hope.

When patients walk through my door for the first time, they have almost all been floundering in illness for years, feeling awful and not knowing what to do about it.

"You're my last hope" is a phrase I hear a lot. Many patients tell me that if this doesn't work, they're ready to give up. That's why it's so important for me to start by reigniting the patient's faith in a brighter future. After all, without hope, there's no survival, as anyone who's survived an ordeal in the wilderness will readily tell you. When Ernest Shackleton, the famous polar explorer, and his crew were stranded for over a year in the Antarctic, it was hope that kept them pushing forward. Without it, why should they continue to fish and hunt? Just for the chance to spend another torturous night in the freezing cold?

But when I say the story gives the patient hope, I don't mean it gives them misguided faith in some miracle drug. Functional medicine isn't about wonder cures or the nutrient of the month. We don't promise patients that this one herb will cure their cancer; if it were that simple, cancer wouldn't kill anyone. The hope I strive to give patients is a faith in their own resilience—a confidence that if they understand the whole picture of their condition, they can confront any situation.

And hope evolves: if a person has cancer and searches for a cure but remains sick, it doesn't mean they give up hope. They can still hope for dignity in death; they can hope to repair their relationships before they go; they can hope for spiritual healing rather than physical healing. In telling a person his story, I never encourage denial or misplaced expectation. I just want my patients to understand the full picture of their illness and remain committed to the journey toward wellness, whatever that means for them.

In the case of Jared, the story inspired hope in him even as the doctrine of traditional medicine caused him to question what I told him. But when he followed what this new functional medicine doctor told him to do, he found that his IBS and his asthma actually started going away. The printed articles from well-regarded medical journals weren't what convinced him; it was the fact that he understood his story, and that when he addressed the problems the story uncovered, he saw marked improvement.

Within a couple of years—during which time he fully recovered—Jared made an important career change: he opened up his own "micro-practice," a practice that was just him, with no nurse or receptionist. He was still working in a hospital to pay the bills, but in his own venture, he was trying something new: healing others through functional medicine.

# Chapter 4

# ASSIMILATION

**Assimilation** (digestion, absorption, microbiota/GI, respiration)

Every living organism exchanges materials with the environment, which includes both permitting needed materials to enter and getting rid of things that are not needed. The physiological system of assimilation encompasses all of the process involved in getting needed inputs into the body, as well as the entry of materials that may not necessarily be needed by the body.

The systems of assimilation includes digestion, the breakdown of food into its component nutrients and non-nutritive substances; absorption, the process of translocating nutrients from "outside" of the body (e.g., the gut) to "inside" it (e.g., the blood); the chemical alteration of substances in the bloodstream by the liver or cellular secretions, which is a major factor in bioavailability; and the entry of those substances into target cells for use in metabolic processes. Gut microbiota play a crucial role in ensuring the integrity of this process in the GI tract.

In addition to the digestion and absorption that occurs in the GI tract, assimilation also includes the entry into the body of substances through other routes, including other mucosa (e.g., respiratory tract, reproductive tract) and across the cutaneous membrane.[2]

When we start training physicians in the field of functional medicine, we start with the fundamentals: assimilation—by far the most critical piece of the matrix I create for my patients. Our bodies are anti-entropy machines, but without assimilation, it would be impossible for us to continue counteracting

---

2   The Institute for Functional Medicine (http://www.functionalmedicine.org).

the body's natural tendency to degrade. And in nearly every patient I see, assimilation is the starting point for recovery.

Assimilation is all about how our bodies take in parts of our environment, break them down into their component pieces, and use those pieces in our system. We carefully prepare about three pounds of this "environment" each day and consume it as food, which is broken down and transferred through the enterocytes—the cells lining the gut wall. Those broken-down bits of food are then efficiently moved into the bloodstream, where our cells absorb and use those nutrients as energy or spare parts to repair damage and generate new cells.

The primary setting for assimilation is the gut. And it turns out the gut has one of the toughest jobs in the body: it houses 70 percent of the immune system and is charged with keeping it running optimally. That's no small responsibility.

One of the gut's biggest challenges is distinguishing between friend and foe. We like to think of our skin as the barrier between us and the outside world, but it's really the gut that distinguishes what is us and what is not us. Elsewhere in the body, organs specialize in either letting nutrients in or keeping toxins out, but not both. The blood-brain barrier, for example—which tightly regulates what gets into the central nervous system from the blood supply—is impermeable to almost anything, as is our skin; organs like the kidneys, on the other hand, are permeable to almost everything. But the gut is unique in that it has to perform both these functions simultaneously. It has to block the bad stuff, and welcome in the good stuff.

As it does its tough sorting work, the gut can make mistakes—and that's where the chain reaction of chronic illness is usually set off. That was the case with one of my patients, a woman named Angela. But Angela didn't come to me for stomach issues, and in the first few minutes I spent with her, I realized it was going to take some work to convince her that the root of her problem was, in fact, assimilation.

●-●-●

I could tell Angela was agitated from the moment I laid eyes on her. A tall woman with stiffly coiffed brown hair, she sat in a chair in the corner of the exam room dressed in a smart business suit. I knew from the questionnaire she'd filled out that she was forty-three.

"How are you today, Angela?" I asked.

"Just fine, thanks. How are you?" She fixed me with bright brown eyes and a quick smile. She was an animated woman, one of those people who fills a room with her energy—yet her aura today wasn't entirely positive. She seemed jumpy and tense.

"I'm great, thanks. What brings you here today?" I asked.

"Well, I've got a bad case of the jimmy legs. It's making me absolutely crazy."

"Jimmy legs?" I asked. I'd never heard the term before.

"Yeah, you know—restless legs." She sat up straight in the chair, not touching the back, and then lifted her feet off the ground and wiggled them back and forth as if she were pedaling a bike. "I've got jimmy legs."

It was hard not to laugh at the sight of this impeccably groomed woman's demonstration. "Tell me more about the jimmy legs," I said.

"Well, it's definitely worst in the evening, especially if I get overtired. It's like I just *have* to move them. I lie in bed for hours trying to get to sleep, and I can't stop them. It's almost like I'm running in place." The agitation in Angela was moving to the fore as she spoke.

"Can you tell me when the last time was that you felt truly well?" I asked— my usual question.

"It's only been happening a couple of months," she replied.

"Okay, good. Any other health problems before that?"

Angela quieted. Her eyes searched my face, as if trying to figure out the trick to my question. "Yes. But they're not related."

"You might be surprised!" I said. "You know what they say. The shin bone's connected to the knee bone and all that."

Reluctantly, she told me she had a history of gastroesophageal reflux disease (GERD, or acid reflux disease). For three years, she'd been on a proton pump inhibitor (PPI)—a type of drug that brings down gastric acid production—to address it. "But it's not a problem," she assured me. "The reflux never bothers me when I'm on my medication. It's like a miracle drug."

After a few more minutes of questioning and filling in the timeline, the next major clue slipped out: "Oh, and I have IBS," Angela told me, looking slightly guilty. "But it's intermittent. It's not really a problem."

"When exactly did the IBS start?" I asked.

Angela crossed her arms. "Does it really matter? How is that relevant?"

They were questions I hear quite frequently. Those of us in medicine have trained our patients to think that everything exists in isolation. From Angela's point of view, she had a single problem, and she wanted to fix it with a medication. From *my* point of view, she was covering bullet holes with Band-Aids. This very efficient, intelligent woman had come in with a specific complaint and was interested in specific answers. But the answer, I knew, lay at the crossroads of several medical specialties. It would take some effort to reveal it.

Unfortunately, Angela didn't seem interested in discussing anything besides the issue she'd come to me for: her restless leg syndrome. It was like talking to Joe Friday—all my inquiries were met with a "just the facts, ma'am," attitude; she was ready to get to the bottom of her very specific complaint, no nonsense. Nevertheless, I kept assuring Angela that ailments as divergent as IBS and jimmy legs could be related. "For one thing," I said, "restless leg syndrome can occur because of a magnesium deficiency, and your proton pump inhibitor can inhibit absorption of minerals. That's just one connection I think is worth exploring."

Angela sighed. "All right, then." She revealed that she was pretty sure she'd always had a sensitive digestive system but that it had worsened recently. "You wouldn't believe how sensitive my stomach is. I've always had to watch what I eat, and if I don't . . . well, let's just say I pay for it big time. It got really bad three years ago, when the reflux stuff started. Then I went on the medicine and it got better, but then two years ago, the IBS kicked in. I can control it pretty well with my diet. I don't eat too much processed food—I try to eat organic, and that works pretty well. But if I go out and have chips and salsa and a big meal . . ."

Unlike some of my patients—including Jared—Angela wasn't on the fearful diet. She wasn't obsessively avoiding certain foods or over-thinking what she ate—she just knew that if she indulged, there was a steep price attached. When Angela's IBS acted up, she'd get constipated for days. Finally, the constipation would crescendo into a horrendous two or three days of stomach cramps and diarrhea, after which the constipation would start to build again. The cycle repeated itself anywhere from once every couple of months to once a week.

By this point, it was clear to me that Angela had some pretty severe GI problems that were almost certainly causing her restless leg syndrome. But I also wanted to get to know Angela more deeply (I'd have to if I was going to convince her of my theory), so I started slipping in a few personal questions here and there.

I found out she was married and had two grown children. One of them had recently had a child of her own, making Angela a grandmother. She never smoked, but did have a couple of drinks most nights to manage her stress.

She'd had the usual childhood illnesses, but nothing of significance. There was no early experience with antibiotics, the factor that had irritated Jared's gut problems. There were no significant toxic exposures either. The one exception was when she'd moved into a new building three or four years back; at first, she was bothered by the pungent smell of brand new carpet and fresh paint. It seemed to be a thing of the past, though—the fumes had dissipated long ago.

But the more I heard about Angela's life, the more I realized how her driven, competitive nature was also affecting her health. She was vice president at a local bank, where the culture was very much of the old boys' club variety. I got the sense that she was trying to outman the men at her bank by putting forth a tough work persona. When I asked what she did for fun, she said, "What do you mean? I don't have fun. I work."

"Well, what do you like to do with your family?" I asked.

"I'm the primary breadwinner. So again," she said crisply, "I work."

Her job pulled her in five different directions at once, and by the end of the day, she was absolutely burnt out. But at bedtime, thoughts of work and her twitchy legs kept her from sleeping. She stayed up late reading and got only about five hours of sleep most nights.

"I still don't get why any of this matters," Angela said after telling me about her patchy sleep patterns. She seemed pretty close to irritated.

I decided to move on. I'd just have to be a little sneaky and circle back later to the personal stuff. By this point, I had prepared her timeline and matrix, and I had a pretty good hunch about how her various GI problems and the restless leg syndrome were related.

I took a deep breath. Story time. "Okay, Angela. Here's what I think is going on. I think you've had this lifelong predisposition to GI sensitivity, in the form of IBS, that escalated toward gastroesophageal reflux disease. Once you got there, you never slowed down long enough to address it. It got progressively worse until you had full-blown reflux and were placed on the proton pump inhibitor, and that PPI just covered it up.

"In fact, even though the PPI helped your reflux in the short term, it can actually make leaky gut worse: PPIs inhibit the acid that normally sterilizes the food you eat, and they also inhibit the absorption of certain nutrients and minerals. That's probably why your irritable bowel syndrome escalated again a year after you started your PPI. Irritable bowel syndrome has further caused difficulties with nutrient absorption, and that's probably why you're now dealing with restless leg syndrome."

Angela was listening closely. Like most of my new patients, she seemed surprised at the depth of my analysis and perhaps a bit skeptical that all these pieces truly fit together. And yet, I could see that she was intrigued.

"So, in order to treat your restless leg syndrome," I continued, "we need to walk this path backwards. We need to understand your lifelong irritable bowel syndrome and whatever resulted in your gastroesophageal reflux. We need to figure out what's going on with your intestinal microflora. We need to fix those and calm down the inflammation in your gut and get you off the PPI so you can start absorbing nutrients better. Once that happens, I'm almost certain your restless legs will start to improve."

Angela, ever fidgety, crossed her arms. "So why the hell haven't any of my other doctors told me this?"

"Because they didn't know. They don't practice functional medicine," I said. "They practice disease management. If you'd gone to another traditional doctor for your restless leg, they would've just scribbled down a prescription for you—one of those drugs where the side effects take up two-thirds of the thirty-second commercial. And if you'd gone to them about your IBS during a constipated period, they probably would've had you taking Miralax every day until you had a bowel movement. If that didn't work, they'd give you a big dose of milk of magnesia."

The prospect didn't seem appealing to Angela.

⬤–⬤–⬤

Fortunately for Angela, I was confident we could save her from that appalling fate. The key to our plan for her would be the five Rs of restoring the gut. Each R represents an integral step toward repairing the body's assimilation function.

- In the **Remove** step, we remove the primary irritant, which is often a dysbiotic bacteria but might also be a harmful medication.

- In the **Replace** step, we substitute the removed element with healthy digestive constituents, perhaps hydrochloric acid or digestive enzymes.

- Then we **Reinoculate** by administering probiotics and prebiotics to rebuild the health population of the gut. (I tell my patients that I use the Carl Sagan approach to gut reinoculation: I use "billions and billions" of probiotics in complex mixtures. That may sound excessive, but there are *trillions* of bacteria in the gut. Adding a few million, which is the standard dose you'll find if you visit the health store, won't do a lot. Most patients need Sagan-level dosage.)

- The **Repair** step is next, and here we administer nutrients—things like glutathione, glutamine, vitamins, and minerals—to address the specific issue with the gut.

- And finally, we **Rebalance**. This step is about understanding what got you to a dysfunctional gut and what you need to do to make sure you don't get back there.

Before Angela left my office after the first visit, I explained what the five Rs would look like for her. We would start by *removing* the PPI that I suspected was causing her trouble. This would likely be her most difficult step, as PPIs are an extremely powerful type of medication. PPIs inhibit proton pumps, as the name suggests, but as the body seeks out the acid these pumps produce, it creates even more of them—even though they remain inhibited by the PPI. But when a patients stops the medication, all those proton pumps become active again, often resulting in significant overproduction of acid. Because of this situation, it takes some time and skill to wean a person off a PPI. Our approach was to switch Angela to a different type of medicine called an H2 blocker while slowly reducing her PPI dosage. We also put her on some natural medicine support for her GI system, including deglycyrrhizinated licorice and zinc-carnosine. We would also *remove* the bad gut bugs with Rifaximin, an antibiotic that isn't absorbed by the body but stays in the gut and is effective at killing off the bad bugs.

We would *replace* the PPI with hydrochloric acid (most people with reflux don't have high acid anyway) and a digestive enzyme. We would *reinoculate* with a Sagan-sized hit of probiotics and a medical food designed to lower inflammation. We would *repair* Angela's gut with nutrients designed to reduce inflammation and heal the gut tissue. And because I suspected that her jimmy legs were the result of magnesium deficiency, I asked her to take a magnesium supplement twice a day.

I stopped when I got to *rebalance*. I'd found Angela to be an amiable, energetic person, but something told me throwing in the lifestyle component (the thing that would ultimately keep her ailments away for good) was too much. Sometimes you only get buy-in after you get results. Instead of giving her any instructions for changing her daily life, I simply made a few observations.

"I think you're a type-A woman, Angela," I said. "A hard-driving businesswoman who's used to pulling herself along by the bootstraps. You don't allow yourself any excuses, and you push yourself hard—probably too hard."

Angela shrugged, stood up, brushed herself off, and thanked me.

I added, "These traits have made you very successful, but they may be adding to your illness. Lets talk more about that next time."

●-●-●

Six weeks later, she was back for her second appointment. Like last time, not a wrinkle could be found on her suit, her hair was pristine, and she still had that vibrant aura.

Angela had experienced minimal improvement in the IBS but had seen pretty good improvement with the acid reflux, even after quitting her PPI. Her jimmy legs, the reason she'd come to me in the first place, had also moderately improved.

But on the visit after that, twelve weeks after I'd met her, Angela was as good as new. Acid reflux, IBS, restless legs—it was all gone.

"I can't believe it!" she said. "I had no idea I could get rid of all of that in less than three months." In her mind, she was cured.

"I'm so excited for you," I said. We chatted a bit more about her newfound wellness before I dropped it on her: "But you're not entirely healed."

She gave me an intense look. "What do you mean? I feel fine."

"Right. That's because you're in temporary remission."

Angela waited for an explanation.

"Well, why do you think you got these things in the first place?" I asked. "Remember how I talked about how you drag yourself by the bootstraps? Remember how I said you pushed yourself too hard?"

Thinking back, Angela nodded.

"Well, are you still doing those things?"

"Yeah. I suppose I am." She shook her head. "But what choice do I have? I don't have the luxury of quitting my job, and I don't think I'd want to even if I did!"

I knew work was important to Angela, and I had no intention of taking that away from her. She was a type-A fighter, and there was nothing wrong with that. She just needed a little yin to complement her yang, unless she wanted to end up sick again.

"Look, you don't have to change who you are at work," I said. "You can still be your ambitious, kinetic self at the bank—but try to turn it off at a certain point each day so you can slow down and enjoy the other areas of your life. I think you're trying to do too much, and it's affecting you negatively."

"How do you mean?" she asked, her eyes narrowing.

"Disease occurs with imbalance, and your chronic stress is probably resulting in imbalanced hormones. Stress increases cortisol, and cortisol can result in insulin resistance. The chain goes on from there: insulin resistance prevents you from burning fat—you burn muscle instead, and the resulting low muscle is associated with poor immune function."

From there, I described for Angela a study my old UCLA professor Norman Cousins had written about, one that I felt emphasized the point that she needed to focus on her lifestyle if she wanted to keep up her newfound health. The study was done with actors, who were brought into the UCLA health center to have their blood drawn. Afterward, they were given an index card with an emotion written on it—*angry, joyous, disappointed, in love*, etc.—and asked to act out that emotion for twenty minutes. After that time had passed, their blood was drawn again. Remarkably, the blood from the second drawing showed very different parameters than the blood drawn twenty minutes before. Actors who'd been acting out negative emotions showed a general decrease in immune function, while positive emotions tended to improve immunity. In some cases, there was as much as a 200 percent difference between the post-acting parameters of the actors assigned the negative emotions and those assigned the positive ones.

"Is that really true?" Angela asked.

I nodded.

She sighed and shook her head, smiling. "All right, then. I'll bite. What do you recommend?"

Angela had told me that she and her husband were very close and that he was always supportive of her busy schedule. I prescribed a simple practice: "When you get home from work, you're going to hug your husband and embrace for one full minute. That is the defining, dividing moment of your day. When you hug him, work is over, and the evening has begun."

Angela smiled dreamily. "That sounds nice."

"The next thing I want you to do is cook dinner together."

Angela laughed. "Okay, I don't think that's going to work. I hate cooking."

"I don't remember asking if you liked cooking," I retorted jokingly. "You need a healthy meal each night and some relaxation. Cooking dinner with your husband is the perfect way to do that. It's about being together, being in charge of what happens in the evening. It's going to be so much better than running back over conversations you had at work or ruminating on an argument with a colleague. Can you do that?"

Angela took a slow, deliberate breath. "If you really think it'll make that big a difference, I'll try."

"Try not!" I croaked, attempting my best Yoda. "Do or do not! There is no try!"

When Angela left my office, I wasn't convinced she'd even get to the point of looking up recipes when she got home. So I was surprised when, a month later at her follow-up, her first words were: "You asshole. I like to cook."

After we had a good laugh, she explained, "I think I hated cooking because I didn't think I had time for it. I wanted to get dinner over with so I could get back to my work. But now Gary and I do the hug and we cook dinner. We talk, we banter. We have a glass of wine. By the time we've eaten, I'm so over work I can't imagine thinking about it."

•-•-•

From there, Angela was on an upward path. Because she was now open to looking at her lifestyle, she was able to ensure she wouldn't easily backslide into disease and discomfort.

Angela still sees me, and the dynamic is totally different. As a new patient, she was a woman on a mission. She wanted her jimmy legs addressed, and that was all. But now we smile and laugh through her appointments—something that's not uncommon in my practice. As people overcome chronic illnesses, their mood lightens noticeably. I tend to run overtime with my long-time patients, often because we're having such a good time laughing and joking. "Sorry to interrupt the party, but you're running behind!" my nurse likes to say when she pops in to keep me on schedule. This transformation happened with Angela—she now asks about my life, and I about hers. Our appointments are relaxed, enjoyable encounters, not grim interrogations.

Perhaps most amazing of all is the last vacation Angela took. She and Gary decided to go to Tuscany on one of those vacations where you spend several days learning from a professional chef. Here was the woman who supposedly hated cooking now choosing to cook on a vacation.

Ultimately, Angela is a perfect example of how three seemingly disparate diagnoses can all be linked to the body's ability to assimilate and utilize nutrients. The first domino to fall had been her gut function, the site of the most important part of assimilation. After that, the spread of disease was helped along by a medicine that partially masked her symptoms. The dominoes just kept falling, until finally she'd ended up with legs so jittery and restless she could hardly sleep at night. But once we struck at the heart of her problem and optimized her gut function, Angela—in a matter of weeks—reached a level of wellness she hadn't experienced in years. She had realized her body's innate capacity to heal.

# Chapter 5

# DEFENSE AND REPAIR

**Defense and Repair** (immune, inflammation, infection/microbiota)

A key element of homeostasis is maintaining a system of defense that prevents entry of pathogens and that removes or incapacitates those that do gain entry. The biological system that we call "defense and repair" includes the innate and adaptive immune mechanisms that have evolved to prevent infection, as well as the repair mechanisms that help restore an injured or infected body to health.

It is well known that the processes used by the immune system can be both a blessing and a curse. When they work as intended, we can avoid illness altogether or recover quickly from an infection. But when the immunologic response to an incursion is overzealous, prolonged, or misplaced, or when these processes occur in the absence of a pathogen, the result can produce major dysfunctions in any or all of the physiological systems.

Inflammation is a key response mechanism in the body's defenses, but it is also an essential prerequisite for initiating the repair process. The inflammatory process starts a cascade of events that activate cellular metabolic and repair mechanisms that enable the body to reestablish homeostasis.[2]

Imagine this: you're standing by a river that's churning with capsized canoes and kayaks. All around, people are flailing and yelling in the water, trying desperately to reach the bank. Instinctively, you and several onlookers dive into the water to pull the unfortunate boaters to shore. Soon, you find ropes and lifesavers and begin using those in the effort, and before long you have a miniature hospital set up, with volunteers attending to the nearly drowned people they've helped rescue. But the problem is, the overturned watercraft just keep coming. The more people you pull out, the more come floating downstream. You labor for hours, exhausting yourself as you devise new ways to bring the swimmers to safety.

But then someone notices the problem: just up the river, there's a waterfall that's causing all the boats to flip. New strategy: you hastily erect a sign upstream warning boaters of the upcoming waterfall. Thanks to the sign, the boaters can divert their craft in time. Because you worked upstream and got to the root cause of the problem, the number of drowning boaters dramatically diminished.

I use that analogy to describe the difference between how conventional medicine and functional medicine approach inflammation. The classic approach is to start downstream, attacking its manifestations with increasingly complex cocktails of drugs. But functional medicine goes upstream. We ask not how we can mitigate a problem short-term, but how we can strike at its core. We try to understand what's triggering the problem—the predisposing genetic factors, the antecedents—and then we figure out the mediators that perpetuate the inflammation. Once we find those triggers, we put the safety on the gun, so to speak, by optimizing the patient's environment through diet and lifestyle.

But first: what exactly *is* inflammation?

We all know its hallmarks—pain, heat, redness, swelling, and loss of function—and when we hear the word itself, most of us conjure up negative thoughts: our swollen lymph nodes in a case of strep throat or the pulsing red tissue around a twisted ankle. As a result, most people think of inflammation as the infection or injury itself, but that's not the case. Inflammation is the body's *response* to insult. It's the effect of your immune system releasing chemicals to fight infection or injury. It's the body's way of defending itself. Without it, we'd be lost.

One of the primary causes of inflammation is the presence of toxins in the body. Any toxin, from heavy metals to PCBs, will cause an inflammatory response. As your white blood cells work to chew up the toxins, they release chemicals that summon other white blood cells to join the effort. Those chemicals are inflammatory, and that's how the process begins.

Trauma causes the same response. When you crush tissue, material from the inside of cells is released—and the body knows that stuff isn't supposed to be out. It is, in essence, just like a toxin. White blood cells are then recruited and brought to the area, and they work to eat up the damaged tissue and make room for new growth. But, again, the chemicals that alert the white blood cells to the problem cause inflammation and its telltale symptoms.

When inflammation serves a short-term purpose, as in response to infection, toxins, or trauma, it's called *acute* inflammation. This is its normal, healthy form. It's the *chronic* type that has earned inflammation its bad reputation.

Chronic inflammation happens when the body is stuck in an inflamed state. The inflammation response is still normal, but it's happening over long periods of time due to a bad combination of environmental inputs in genetic predisposition. When your body is inflamed at a low level for that long, you begin to see major problems creeping up: heart disease, diabetes, arthritis, chronic fatigue syndrome, fibromyalgia, and a host of other diagnoses no one wants to receive.

Chronic inflammation even causes afflictions of a cognitive and psychological nature. Thanks to the blood-brain barrier, the brain has a segregated immune system and is generally protected from most of the stuff going on in the body. However, chronic inflammation can activate the brain's immune system, which can lead, over time, to problems like depression, ADHD, and dementia. There's no question: an inflamed brain is not a happy brain.

Compounding the problem, inflammation can affect the brain through another mechanism: the inflammatory chemicals used to summon the white blood cells. These chemicals have psychoactive effects and are small enough to penetrate the blood-brain barrier. When they do, they give you that terrible sick feeling—the one that makes you say, "I feel so awful I just want to die" when you only have a cold. At lower but persistent levels, these chemicals may make you feel constantly irritable, tired, and gloomy.

Chronic inflammation—the equivalent of a long-term war raging inside you—can also lead to autoimmunity. In any war, you're going to get attrition: you're going to run out of supplies and spare parts, while fatigue and weakness can even lead to tragic friendly fire. In a chronically inflamed state, your body's ability to repair itself will suffer, and it is more and more likely to attack its own tissue inadvertently.

Unfortunately, when a person goes to a traditional doctor with an inflammation-related problem, the physician will typically treat the symptom but ignore the root cause—a method diametrically opposed to a functional medicine approach.

◉—◉—◉

When Carey first came to my office, she was fifty-six, but she looked at least five or six years older than that. Her eyes had a sunken look, set in two dark circles. She was thin but didn't look healthy, and her motion was slow and deliberate. Like many of my patients, she came in on a referral from someone else I was treating.

"I'm here for my rheumatoid arthritis," Carey told me. "My doctor wants to put me on Enbrel, but that doesn't seem like a good idea to me, especially after I read the booklet."

I had to agree with her. Enbrel, an arthritis drug designed to kill off the part of the immune system that is attacking the patient's body, has an ominous litany of possible side effects. Yet, Carey's pain had advanced to the point that she didn't know what else to do. The knotted, slightly misshapen hands folded in her lap were evidence of her struggle.

"I was diagnosed with the arthritis about . . . fifteen years ago," Carey continued flatly. "I was about forty. I started getting really stiff in my joints, and then it became pain and swelling. They did a rheumatoid arthritis panel and diagnosed me; then they put me on Celebrex"—a nonsteroidal anti-inflammatory drug. "That helped for a little bit, but then after . . . I'd say a year, it got worse, and I went to a rheumatologist."

"And he prescribed you the methotrexate?" I asked, glancing down at her file. Methotrexate was a drug originally developed for chemotherapy but later commonly used to treat arthritis.

"Yes. I take that every week still, but even now, it isn't working. He added Plaquenil after six months or so. So now I take all three, and I get steroids when I have a flare-up. Quite a cocktail, I suppose." Carey laughed, but her smile didn't reach her eyes. Though she was trying hard to seem jovial, her heart wasn't in it.

"But you're still hurting, right?"

"I am. That's why I'm here. I don't know what else to do except go on the Enbrel."

From there, we dove into Carey's past, and I began working on her timeline and matrix. Like so many patients, she seemed guarded and a little confused as to why I wasn't writing out a list of the herbs that would make her pain go away. But I explained what functional medicine was all about—connections, root causes, lifestyle—and we moved on.

How chronic inflammation manifests itself in your health depends on your genetic susceptibility. In one person, chronic inflammation may cause trouble in the bowels; in another, it may hasten along complications from heart disease. And some people are genetically predisposed to inflammation itself. That seemed to be the case for Carey. She told me her mother suffered from rheumatoid arthritis, too, and that she had an aunt with lupus. A different aunt had been diagnosed with Grave's disease, or autoimmune thyroiditis.

However, here's an important side note: **genes do not equal destiny**. The way your genes act is always a complex interplay between predisposition and environment, and the good news is that you can change one of those factors. Although genes are fixed, they are constantly interacting with everything around us—the food we eat, the air we breathe, the stress we feel. By manipulating the environment, we can turn one set of genes on and another set off. I know it sounds strange, but it's true: a change in lifestyle can alter which portions of your DNA are active and which aren't. That means that by living your life in a new way, you can literally become a different person.

When I asked Carey to tell me about the last time she felt truly well, she said it had been during her thirties. "I was a bit of a health nut, actually. I ate well—tons of vegetables and fruits and fish. I worked out and did yoga. I felt really healthy."

"So what happened?" I asked. "Why don't you do all that anymore?"

"Well . . . ," she said cautiously, "I went through a lot around forty."

"What happened?"

"I don't know. I don't want to whine. A lot of personal stuff."

"Hmm. I think we should talk about that," I said.

"I just feel like I'll be complaining."

"Carey, when we're in this room, there's no such thing as complaining. You're telling me about your life, and I'm trying to understand what bearing it's had on your health. I have to understand your history; it's that simple. You are *not* complaining!"

Though I had to remind her of that a couple more times, Carey eventually opened up about the circumstances that directly preceded her arthritis diagnosis. Her adult son had been killed in a car accident. She was absolutely devastated. Then, in the aftermath of the tragedy, her marriage started to disintegrate. She and her husband—a financial analyst at a big corporation, a high-end executive kind of guy—simply couldn't work through their grief and stay in the marriage. Because of the split, Carey was to move. She went from living in a big house on the lake in an outer suburb of Minneapolis to living in an apartment by herself—and it wasn't a luxurious apartment, either. The change in her support system, and in herself, hit her hard. Under the massive load of her grief and the demise of her relationship, her self-esteem had also faltered. Like many of us, her self-esteem was tied up in the wrong things: her children, her house, her lifestyle, and her status.

These devastating circumstances had broken her. She felt as though her life had imploded. She was depressed and suffered from ongoing anxiety. On top of it all, her financial future seemed bleak; a stay-at-home mom while her kids were at home, she didn't have a career to augment her resources after the divorce. Carey's health habits evaporated, replaced by a new junk-food habit, a lapsed gym membership, and long nights in front of the TV. As the same time, she fell out of her social circle. Within a year of the divorce, she was at the doctor, getting her prescription for Celebrex. Fifteen years later, she was still suffering as a result of a poor lifestyle and a festering pile of negative emotions. Her now-dulled grief at the loss of her son was interwoven with great resentment for her ex-husband, who had since moved on to a younger second wife.

"I lost my life, but he still has his," Carey said. The firm set of her jaw told me she was truly angry. "He's as happy as ever. But I worked just as hard as he did. I made us as successful as we were. I am the one with the people skills. I was the networker. Why is he the one over there living the high life?"

"That has to make you mad."

"Of course it does," she snapped, unleashing some of her pent-up ire on me.

"And it should. That's a bad situation. But you know, we are one being. We often think of ourselves as several distinct entities—a body, mind, and spirit—but we aren't. We are one. The totality of you is the result of all of your thoughts, beliefs, foods, activities, associations, friendships . . . all of it and more, and the way you process them. Life is like a pinball machine. We get hurled out of the canon and start bouncing off of things. Each of those *ding, ding, dings!* is an experience that shapes us. Our lives are the often-unconscious summation of all of those experiences.

"Have you ever read or heard about the mother of a child who was murdered who then goes on to befriend the murderer? How can that happen? How can that be? Forgiveness. Forgiveness is not about forgiving the perpetrator, it is about moving past the events. Forgiveness is for you. Forgiveness does not mean you think what happened is okay. Forgiveness means you no longer give it power over you. The events that have happened in your life still have power over you. We need to explore that and learn from it. These feelings are hurting you from the inside, and they're making your physiological problems worse. It's about letting go of your anger, because it's not going to help you feel better. Let's find ways to be done with this."

Carey nodded but didn't say anything.

By now, I felt that I had a good picture of Carey's situation, so I moved on to her story. "All right, Carey. Let's go back over everything, and I'll explain what I think is happening based on our discussion. First, it appears to me that you are experiencing the normal response to a mismatch between your environment and your genes. It looks to me as though you carry this genetic predisposition for inflammation, but you managed it very well for a long time. Maybe it was because of watching your mother's health struggles that you chose to have the healthy lifestyle you did in your thirties. Maybe you weren't specifically trying to, but you kept your inflammation under control through your diet and exercise.

"But then you had a major upheaval in your life—several major upheavals. Your entire lifestyle changed abruptly—and, unfortunately, in a way that was pro-inflammatory. So you're no longer taking in as many anti-inflammatory nutrients as you were, and you're taking in more pro-inflammatory nutrients. Plus, your thoughts and emotions, your psychic turmoil, are just promoting the inflammation. Over time, that's taken its toll and unmasked your genetic predisposition for inflammation. That constant, low-level inflammation turned up as arthritis."

I paused, waiting for Carey's reaction. She was nodding, looking defeated.

"So, the good news: here's our plan. We need to find as many triggers and mediators as we can, and rematch your diet and lifestyle to your genetic predispositions. When we calm those down, you're going to see a lot of improvement."

As I do with many patients, I put her on "Dr. Sult's Magic Formula," which consists of our elimination diet, anti-inflammatory medical food, a dose of anti-inflammatory fish oil, and high-dose probiotic and immune support. We also ordered lab tests and planned to review them upon her return.

When Carey left that day, she still seemed subdued and upset. But by the time she came back for her next visit six weeks later, she was already feeling better. She was still on all her medications, but the stiffness and pain had relented slightly. When we looked over her lab tests together, we saw that she also had some issues in the gut: a lot of indigestion and irritable bowel kind of stuff. She also had low omega-3 fatty acids, high trans-fatty acids, and high omega-6 fatty acids—especially a pretty destructive one called arachidonic acid. Thanks to her lifestyle, Carey was flooded with harmful toxins and chronically inflamed. My Magic Formula had shoved her in the right direction, but if we were going to make any progress toward wellness, we had to give Carey an oil change.

●-●-●

No matter what form your chronic inflammation has taken, there are a few simple steps you can take to reduce it and thus begin to counteract the downstream effects. Here are the four pillars of keeping your inflammation under control, all of which I covered with Carey.

**1. Eat a variety of naturally colorful foods, in abundance.** To lessen unhealthy inflammation, shoot for a colorful diet—preferably without using Skittles (although each Skittle *does* contain a full day's supply of artificial food coloring). In natural food, color generally means phytonutrients. Avoid white things—think flour, potatoes, or sugar—and go for color: yellow peppers, bright red radishes, deep-green spinach, shiny purple eggplant. If you're choosing between a white potato and a yellow yam, go for the yam.

The second piece is variety. So many of my patients say, "Yeah I eat vegetables—I have peas and carrots and corn, and then I have peas and carrots and corn, and then sometimes I have peas and carrots and corn." Well, that's not much in the way of variety. If you think about the minimum of five fruits and vegetables a day, that's thirty-five fruits and vegetables in a week. I challenge you to consume thirty-five *different* fruits and vegetables in a week. Some patients ask, "Are there even thirty-five different kinds of fruits and vegetables?" (The answer is yes, by the way.) I tell them to see how close they can come—the goal is to be creative, to look around the produce section or the farmers' market with fresh eyes, and think, *Oh yeah! I forgot about that one!* or *Hmm, I wonder what that one tastes like* . . . The more variety the better, and the more color the better.

As part of her elimination diet, I also encouraged Carey to consume plenty of foods higher in omega-3s and lower in omega-6s, especially the longer omega-6s like arachidonic acid (found in foods like red meat, organ meat, dairy, and pork). We eliminated trans fats from her diet and put her on more antioxidants: plenty of cumin, rosemary, and fish oil. I knew all these would work together to reduce her inflammation.

**2. Eat fish at least a couple of times a week.** Getting plenty of fish in the diet is another effective way to combat chronic inflammation. I pressed upon Carey the importance of eating fish at least twice a week but warned her about avoiding large predator fish, which are more likely to be contaminated with mercury. When choosing between types of fish, always go smaller and further down the food chain, as the smaller fish are less likely to accumulate chemicals and toxins. Pick sockeye, pollack, or orange roughy over king salmon.

**3. Reduce toxic exposure at home and at work.** I encouraged Carey to use nontoxic cleaning products and nontoxic toiletries. I had her buy a water filter for her kitchen and air filters for her living room and bedroom. I told her to refrain from spraying any chemical-laden junk in her home or on her yard, and I also put her on a probiotic and immune support.

**4. Engage in joyous activity.** When it comes to exercise, joyous activity is better than forced activity. If you are going to work out, find something you enjoy doing. For example, if you find dancing more fun than riding a stationary bike, take dance classes. And if you don't have a partner, give Zumba a try. If you have the will to exercise, you'll find a way, and it will be a lot easier if you make it something you enjoy, not something you dread.

"Joyous activity" doesn't just have to be exercise, though—it can be anything that you feel meaningful, productive, and happy doing. To find meaningful activity, follow causes you care about—see if you can volunteer or, in some active way, support a cause that's important to you.

The varied nature of these steps illustrates the complex interconnectedness of the matrix. Although we are talking about inflammation, interventions in three other matrix sectors (assimilation, biotransformation and elimination, and the psychosocial/spiritual realm) can help manage it.

Back when I first met Carey, I couldn't help but notice the trouble she had standing from the exam-room chair as she prepared to leave. She rocked back and forth to build momentum and then, with great effort and an audible groan, pushed herself to her feet.

"You know what Sophia Loren said about aging, right?" I'd said to Carey, smiling.

"I don't think so," she replied.

"Well, you know she's a bombshell, a sex symbol, and this reporter once asked about her secret to staying so graceful and beautiful. She said, 'Never groan when you stand up.'"

Carey and I shared a laugh as I walked her back toward the waiting area and the front door, and then she was off.

Over the next three years, we didn't get Carey off of methotrexate, and it took a while to get her off of the Plaquenil. And yet we won: because we went upstream to address the inflammation, she reduced her pain enough that she didn't have to go on Enbrel—her main concern. Today, she is largely pain-free, and she's also reduced the dosage on her methotrexate and stopped taking prednisone. She still has the slight deformity in her hands—nothing will change that—but it's no longer getting worse. She doesn't feel like she's deteriorating day by day anymore. And thanks to the reduction in pain, she can do almost anything she wants with her hands. I'm still hopeful that, in the future, we'll be able to wean Carey off all her drugs, but for now, she is happy and continues to improve. She's more engaged with life, her memory has improved, and—though I'm not *necessarily* saying low inflammation will get you this kind of attention—she even has a new flame.

Functional medicine isn't about handing out wonder cures to everyone; it's about doing the best we can for each individual. If a person just needs lifestyle modification, that's great. But sometimes they do need medicine or surgery, and we support that. We just want to manage illness in the least invasive way possible and to address causes, not symptoms. I suppose I could write a book of only my "wonder cases" (it would be like most books in the genre), and I do have many stories of astounding recoveries, but to tell only those feels untrue, unbelievable. I want you to see truth, not exaggeration. Not every case is a home run. But you can win the game with base hits. Carey had a triple.

To an outside observer, Carey today looks much like she did when she walked into my practice several years ago. But if you knew Carey before, you can identify the change. She has a sparkle in her eyes, and her smile is genuine. When she laughs, it doesn't sound like a cover-up. She enjoys life again.

Over the years, she's been able to come to grips with her son's death, and she's let go of some of the anger surrounding her divorce and her financial circumstance; I think that's been a major contributor to her pain management and reduced inflammation. Of course, changing her relationship with her own emotions was an improvement in its own right. But creating a healthier relationship with these emotions also helped her regain control and prevented her from pulling the biological triggers of inflammation over and over, every day. Without inflammation-inducing chemicals flooding her bloodstream, the world seemed like a better place.

Carey also consciously decided that a healthy diet was going to be her hobby, just as it had been when she was in her healthy thirties or cooked dinner for her family. She took classes and made regular trips to Minneapolis's best culinary stores, if for no other reason than to be with other people interested in cooking. She found herself making new friends this way. Before long, she was preparing delicious, balanced meals in her own kitchen—something she hadn't done regularly since leaving her husband. She got in the habit of making big meals twice a week, and the leftovers were enough to feed her on the days she cooked more lightly. The sense of control this gave her, the sense of doing something positive for herself, was every bit as good for her as the food she was preparing. Carey came to a recent appointment wearing a T-shirt that said "No junk food tastes as good as wellness feels. EAT WELL, BE WELL."

At the end of her fourth or fifth visit with me, Carey reminded me of the Sophia Loren story I'd told her.

"It just resonated with me somehow," she said. "I decided it was my life's mission to not be a person who groans when she stands up. And look at this." Beaming a genuine smile, Carey propelled herself out of her chair—no rocking, and not a hint of a groan.

# Chapter 6

# ENERGY

**Energy** (energy regulation, mitochondrial function)

As defined by physicists, energy is the capacity to do work, i.e., to make something change. The physiological system of energy encompasses this ability from the molecular level all the way up to the organismal and ecological levels and beyond.

At the subcellular level, energy is produced by the mitochondria, which capture energy liberated from the breakdown of nutrients and transform it into the coenzyme adenosine triphosphate (ATP), which is closely involved in energy transfer. This highly controlled process requires the coordination of hundreds of metabolites; imbalances in the levels of these metabolites create energy deficits for the cell. When such energy imbalances occur in cells, it can affect the function of tissues, organs, or indeed the entire organism.

While mitochondria are the main producers of energy in the body, they are not the whole energy story. The way that energy is consumed in the body creates electrical fields that can be evaluated (e.g., EEG, ECG) that are external manifestations of internal body processes that can serve both as markers of body function (or dysfunction) and as signals to other nearby organisms. At the organismal/ecological level, this energy pattern, while little used in conventional Western medicine, has been recognized for thousands of years by other medical models and is variously referred to as Qi, Prana, and Pneuma; it is thought to affect other organisms and the environment. Medicine that seeks to intervene at this higher level of energy "flow" is sometimes referred to as energy medicine.[2]

On the morning after Easter of 1987, Greg LeMond—winner of the previous year's Tour de France—walked out onto a large ranch in northern California, accompanied by his uncle and brother-in-law. The three carried shotguns. They were off to bag a turkey or two.

Hours later, Greg lay bleeding on the ground, gasping for breath. His brother-in-law, mistaking him for a turkey, had fired his twelve-gauge at Greg through some bushes. Forty pellets ripped open his back and side. One lung collapsed, and two pellets became lodged in the lining of his heart. He would lose 65 percent of his blood.

Thanks to the hasty arrival of a helicopter—and Greg's youth and fitness—he survived, but there was no question that he'd miss the upcoming Tour de France. Within a couple of years, however, he was back in top form, retaking the championship at the world's top cycling race in both 1989 and 1990.

And yet, after those two victories, LeMond's physical ability deteriorated quickly. He showed great exhaustion and struggled to finish races. By 1994, he announced his retirement, citing a condition most Americans hadn't heard of: mitochondrial myopathy.

"I can't spell it," Greg told the *New York Times* upon his retirement, "but I can say it's dysfunctional mitochondria, which won't help me produce energy. My energy-delivery system has been off whack."[3] Due to these dysfunctional mitochondria, the former cycling champion was suffering from symptoms much like those of a muscular disease.

Mitochondria—subcellular units often referred to as "the powerhouses of the cell"—are a vital part of the process that supplies the body with energy. And our bodies, those anti-entropy machines that are constantly trying to create order from disorder, need plenty of energy. Greg LeMond's is an extreme case, but when any of us encounter trauma with long-term effects, especially in tandem with a second or third trauma, our mitochondria can become taxed, creating an energy deficit. Suddenly our bodies no longer have what it takes to keep up.

LeMond's mitochondrial weakness manifested itself in the muscles and was thus termed "mitochondrial *myopathy*" (*myo* is Greek for "muscle"), but the word "mitochondriopathy" refers to a broader set of dysfunctions that can affect nearly every aspect of health, from digestion to cognitive function. The common link is the same: a disturbance in the energy section of the matrix.

---

3    Samuel Abt, "Greg LeMond Ending Career," *New York Times*, December 3, 1994.

When Dan came to my office, he was in a downward spiral. He was a fifty-eight-year-old electrical engineer who worked for a big company in California, and he'd been a rising star in his field earlier in his career, quickly ascending the corporate ladder. He'd first landed a position as manager of his department and soon thereafter became manager of an entire division of the company. But in recent years, Dan had noticed that work was more difficult. He was making silly mistakes and struggling to keep up. His charmed career would be facing its first big roadblock if he didn't figure out a way to improve his performance.

Dan came to his appointment with his wife, Rebecca, and I was immediately struck by how somber they both seemed. Their interlinked fingers kept them connected, but both of their gazes were turned toward me with a look I recognized: wary hope. I pulled up a chair for Rebecca and began to ask Dan about what brought him here.

"At first, I just thought I wasn't as sharp as I used to be," Dan told me. "I'd forget about meetings or neglect details here and there. Not a big deal."

The problems got progressively worse, though.

"Pretty soon, I was struggling to learn our new systems, and now I feel like I'm dropping every other ball that's tossed my way," he said. As Dan told me about his work troubles, his face was grave, and he spoke hesitatingly. During his frequent pauses, Rebecca chimed in, filling in a detail or encouraging him to elaborate.

"Sometimes I wonder how big a problem this really is," Dan said at one point with a shrug. "In the old days, when I was an engineer, I was trained in analog. Digital didn't exist, and I never really learned it."

Immediately, alarm bells rang: Dan was confabulating. In other words, he was not lying but instead telling an internally consistent story that he hoped would explain away his deficit. Dan was a smart guy, and over the years, he'd learned how to cover up his impairment with this type of confabulation. But his excuse about not understanding digital systems didn't make sense to me—he worked in a semiconductor industry, for Pete's sake! Surely he understood digital technology to some degree. Plus, his main job now was managing people.

I looked him in the eye. "I'm not sure I'm buying this."

"Excuse me?"

"Dan, the story you're telling me is that you were a rising star in this organization. That leads me to believe that you were the go-getter in school and mastered new concepts quickly. Now you're saying that the shift from analog to digital is too much for you? That's just not consistent."

Rebecca looked startled and glanced between the two of us, ready to intervene. But Dan just sighed. "Yeah. You're right."

"We call it confabulation," I said. "You're unconsciously creating a false history to serve your own purposes. You've used this excuse to explain to your boss—and yourself—why you're struggling at the job, but it doesn't seem like your job has much to do with engineering. You're a manager. The excuse doesn't really make sense."

Dan nodded his assent. Clearly, he'd come to see me because he felt something was wrong enough for him to be there, but he was struggling to give up the story of his supposedly insufficient engineering background. His actions were contradictory, but that's human nature. We tell ourselves what we want to believe. Fortunately, his ability to reason was intact enough that he understood what he was doing.

The problem started over a decade ago. Ten years before he came to me, Dan had gone to his primary care physician about the frustrating lack of mental acuity he was experiencing. The doctor had put him through the usual routine, giving him a mini–mental status exam—a thirty-point questionnaire used to screen for cognitive impairment—and running some blood tests. "You're fine, Dan," the physician had told him at the follow-up visit. "You're in your late forties. You're getting older. Memory issues are a fact of life."

But the mental sluggishness continued to be a thorn in Dan's side. "Used to be, everything was a snap of the fingers," he said. "But now I go to work, doing the same thing I've done for twenty years, and I have to sit there and think about every little thing I do for ten minutes. I can't figure out even simple problems sometimes."

Dan's fear regarding his deteriorating mental abilities had been confirmed soon after the doctor told him not to worry: after a series of serious mistakes, Dan's boss demoted him. I could tell this part of the story was especially hard for Dan to tell. He crossed his arms, got stiff, stared at the floor.

"It was humiliating," Dan said quietly. "After that, I decided I needed a second opinion, so I went to the University of San Francisco Medical Center. They ran a lot of tests. They did a brain scan and a lumbar puncture . . . and they told me it was Alzheimer's."

I had scanned Dan's questionnaire before the appointment and knew about the devastating diagnosis he'd received. Nevertheless, the word *Alzheimer's* hung in the air of the exam room. Both Dan and Rebecca looked dismayed, close to terrified. Both had tears in their eyes.

Dan cleared his throat. "And now on top of this, I'm thinking I'm going to get demoted again."

"What gives you that feeling?" I asked.

"After all the things I've been screwing up, my bosses don't look at me the way they used to. They don't trust me, and I don't blame them. I feel like I'm in a free fall. I don't want to end up in a year sitting in some hospital with my head tipped to the side, drooling. But that's where it feels like I'm heading."

As he spoke, his eyes began to glisten. There was an uncomfortable silence, and Rebecca leaned closer to him so that they were shoulder to shoulder, hands still connected and resting on Dan's thigh.

"Excuse me a moment," Dan said. He patted Rebecca's hand, stood, and walked into the hallway, pulling the door shut behind him.

Rebecca pursed her lips and blinked hard. I could tell from the resolute set of her jaw that she had steeled herself for whatever was going to happen to her husband—but if there was a chance to fight, she would take it.

"Dan never gets emotional like this," she said softly. "He's your typical stoic Minnesotan. The man I know would've sat here and talked to you matter-of-factly about what was going on, even if it was Alzheimer's. I don't know how else to say this, but that's not the man I know."

For both of them, Dan's problems had become a huge emotional liability. Beyond simply worrying about the deterioration of his health, Rebecca was terrified that she was losing her husband and best friend day by day. And the situation was no better for Dan, of course, who felt like he was slowly losing himself. He was experiencing something common among people with dementia: the slow deterioration of executive control in the brain and, along with it, an increase in raw, hard-to-control emotions.

◆-◆-◆

Any physician will tell you they get at least one person a day who comes in concerned about memory impairment, and that all these patients have one main fear: Alzheimer's. Fortunately, in the majority of cases, it isn't Alzheimer's.

Alzheimer's disease isn't a clear-cut or tangible condition. It's a biochemical process in the brain, and we don't understand it well. The question I wanted to get at with Dan was, what would cause these biochemical impairments? I knew one possibility was that his mitochondria were struggling to provide his brain with the energy it needed to function in top form. It was possible that, like Greg LeMond, Dan's trouble could be traced back to problems in his cellular powerhouses.

Ideally, your body, with the help of the mitochondria, should be producing thirty-eight molecules of ATP—the coenzyme often referred to as the currency of molecular energy transfer—per molecule of glucose. But when the mitochondria break down and perform ineffectively, as in mitochondriopathy, you may be producing twenty-eight ATP molecules instead of thirty-eight, or maybe you're only producing fifteen. Your energy efficiency drops, and you might not be able to efficiently make hormones, build proteins, or repair DNA. You often feel lethargic and fatigued. It's like running a fancy sports car when two cylinders are out.

So how do mitochondria malfunction in the first place and cause this subpar performance? Here's the short answer: mitochondriopathy is typically the result of trauma. LeMond's trauma was clear: the violent hunting accident that had riddled him with metal pellets, followed by competition at the elite level. But in most people, mitochondrial problems come from a combination of two or more less-dramatic traumas, generally in combination with a genetic predisposition (in other words, an antecedent). Perhaps one person has worked a stressful job for ten years, eaten a poor diet, and been in a serious car accident. Perhaps another person had two major operations in one year. It's in compounded situations like these that most people get out of balance—their bodies have a tremendous demand for the repair and rebuilding of tissue. All that stress and injury requires massive detoxification, and it is through the process of detoxification that mitochondria often run into trouble.

This is one of countless examples of how the areas of the matrix overlap and interrelate, in this case the energy sector and the assimilation and biotransformation sectors, the latter of which handles the breaking down and elimination of toxins. The detoxification process (which we'll discuss in more depth in the following chapter) involves two phases. In very simple terms, phase one converts toxins to "reactive intermediates," and phase two finishes the job and eliminates the intermediates.

The problem is that when a person is nutritionally depleted, phase one detoxification pathways get all revved up and create abundant reactive intermediaries, including free radicals, but then the body doesn't have the nutritional resources to carry out phase two. When that happens, free radicals—atoms or molecules with unpaired electrons—accumulate in the body. Think of a funnel: when phase one is working fine, it's like pouring free radicals into the wide top end, but as phase two fails, it's as if the outlet to the funnel shrinks; when free radicals go in faster than they're able to come out, they back up and eventually overflow into the body. These free radicals are highly chemically reactive and damage the body over time. (I once had a professor who said that free radicals are promiscuous molecules: they want an electron and they'll take it from anywhere they can get it.) Mitochondria, busy at work creating energy, are especially sensitive to such injury, even though they created the free radicals in the first place. The mitochondria, full of free radicals, are like a buzzing high-voltage power line after a morning rain, charged with potentially harmful electricity.

Mitochondria, by the very nature of their work, make free radicals constantly. But when phase two detoxification breaks down due to the stress of the double-trauma (or triple-trauma) scenario, the mitochondria become overwhelmed. Under the toxic burden from injury or accident, they are no longer able to defend themselves from the free radicals they're making. Suddenly the body is producing far fewer than its goal of thirty-eight ATP molecules per glucose molecule, and your energy efficiency plummets, which can lead to a host of other problems.

Of course, it's important to remember that inflammation, detoxification, and free radicals are all part of the body's normal, healthy response to its environment. Most of the time, the body deals with injury in a closed feedback loop: inflammation begets anti-inflammation begets normal healthy tissue. Stubbing your toe usually isn't going to lead to mitochondriopathy. The problem happens when a susceptible person experiences repeated traumas that lead to a "feed-forward" loop, where inflammation begets more inflammation begets more inflammation. That happens when a person is out of balance—or, as a practitioner of functional medicine would say, when the genetic milieu of the patient is mismatched with his environment.

This mitochondrial trouble manifests itself in many ways, including the Alzheimer's-like symptoms with which Dan was struggling. Even if you suffer from a less extreme condition, especially one that causes tiredness, muscle pain, or brain fog (perhaps fibromyalgia, chronic fatigue syndrome, polymyalgia rheumatics), you almost certainly have an issue with energy and mitochondria. Once you determine that the assimilation area of the matrix is in good shape, the energy area is the next place you'll want to look to start solving these problems. That's not to give precedence to assimilation over energy: in truth, every area of the matrix—in fact, every aspect of simple well-being—is dependent on the ability to make energy.

◉-◉-◉

After a couple of minutes, Dan composed himself and came back into the exam room. His eyes glinted, and he took his seat beside Rebecca without looking at her.

"Here's the problem with Alzheimer's disease," I said before we started the timeline. "It isn't something you can cut out of your body and lay on the table and say, 'See, that's your Alzheimer's disease!' We don't understand the condition that well, so we should start by looking for any underlying issues you have that could be contributing to these cognitive problems. The end diagnosis of Alzheimer's may just be the patterns that a particular set of inflammatory conditions has led to."

After a long pause, Dan said, "I'm not sure I understand what you mean."

"When I was in medical school," I explained, "we were told that the brain doesn't heal. Now we know it does heal, but it heals extremely slowly. We know that you have injury to your brain, but the problem is we don't know which part of your brain has to be rebuilt and which part is just stunned and can come back more quickly. Hopefully we'll find that out."

They both seemed game to move forward, but Rebecca nodded along with particular enthusiasm. She was terrified, I could tell, of watching her husband slip away. "Are you saying we can . . . cure his Alzheimer's?"

"No, not exactly," I said, quick to align her expectations with reality. "I can't say whether the brain will heal or not. What I am saying is that we need to explore this situation and see if we can find a process to improve that might halt the deterioration or perhaps heal some of the damage over time. But that doesn't mean we can give him some supplements and cure it."

Rebecca, her enthusiasm tempered, said, "That's fine. We understand. We just want to do everything we can."

Dan didn't have a clear "not well since" moment—he described a slow, steady decline, but he couldn't put a finger on when it had started. He'd had the flu a couple of times, occasional aches and pains throughout his body. Nothing was leaping out at me until he started telling me about his family.

"We've got two sons and two daughters," Dan said, "and we're pretty outdoorsy. I hunt with my son, Zach, and we go on canoe trips. Camping trips. Things like that. We've got a cabin where we go for summers."

He then described the location of the cabin—and placed it right in the middle of an area known to be highly endemic for deer ticks, which can carry Lyme disease. Given that he was there every summer for many weeks of vacation away from their current home in the Bay Area, and was outdoors most of that time, could exposure to Lyme disease have been the trigger for his mental decline?

Certainly, chronic Lyme disease—a long-term bacterial colonization that causes continuous inflammatory reactions in the body—puts stress on the detoxification process and, thus, increases harmful free radicals as the mitochondria go full blast. The resultant mitochondriopathy could have manifested in Dan's brain. (Of course, if you have inflammation or Lyme disease, you're not necessarily going to get Alzheimer's—it's the combination of genetic predisposition, trigger, mediators, and the location of the major injury.)

Chronic Lyme disease is a controversial diagnosis. The Infectious Diseases Society of America will tell you it doesn't exist, despite abundant evidence to the contrary; the International Lyme and Associated Disease Society has done a good job of compiling the data about this chronic condition. But regardless of the controversy, I felt that given Dan's background, this was the most likely cause of the inflammation and mitochondrial breakdown that had caused the symptoms of Alzheimer's.

By the time we'd filled out Dan's matrix and gone through how his conditions interacted with each other, he and his wife looked worn out. I explained that Alzheimer's disease is associated with a lot of inflammation in the brain and that at the very least, we needed to do whatever we could do to manage inflammation in Dan's brain. I also explained that because of his significant exposure to ticks that carry Lyme disease, I felt we should investigate the possibility that the chronic form of this condition was contributing to his difficulties. I shook Dan's hand and gave Rebecca a hug, assuring them that we'd get to the bottom of it.

●-●-●

Over the next few weeks, we did a bunch of tests on Dan. One was called a NutrEval, which measures nutritional efficiency, and we found that he had problems with the utilization of certain B vitamins and antioxidants. On Dan's initial standard testing for Lyme disease, the results came back normal. This didn't rule Lyme disease out, though—this test relied on the immune system's antibodies to detect the condition, but people with Lyme disease often have what we call an "immune blind spot." The second test we did was a culture, where the bugs are actually grown from a blood sample. Dan got a culture done at a specialty lab, and the results came back positive.

To treat the chronic Lyme disease, we put Dan on multiple antibiotics, which he ended up staying on for four years. But the other pieces of Dan's treatment can benefit anyone's mitochondrial health and energy efficiency and help insulate you from the myriad problems that can be exacerbated by mitochondriopathy.

First, we started with the basics and put Dan on a diet that was high in fruits and vegetables. When you're eating a variety of fruit and vegetables, you're benefiting from phytonutrients that help with detoxification (and thus reduce the load your mitochondria carry). In addition to giving Dan some medical foods, we also discussed how he could work more anti-inflammatory herbs and antioxidant-boosting foods into his eating routine.

Second, we wanted to put Dan on B vitamin and antioxidant supplements, since the NutrEval test had shown he had trouble utilizing these. Also, B vitamins are particularly important to the energy-producing activity of the cells. For a great source of these vitamins, look for a broad-spectrum multivitamin with lots of antioxidants.

Finally, we encouraged Dan to get plenty of the nutrients that we know are important in mitochondria functioning, like folic acid, coenzyme Q10 (CoQ10), lipoic acid, and PQQ, a specific nutrient that helps you actually make new mitochondria. To get him those nutrients, we gave him a CoQ10 supplement— available in most pharmacies and grocery stores—at 200 milligrams two times a day. He took the lipoic acid supplement at 400 milligrams two times a day, and PQQ at 40 milligrams two times a day; both of these are widely available as well. Dan also consumed Dynamic Greens, a "super green food," to boost his phytonutrition. Finally, he took large doses of probiotics—100 billion—two times a day and IgG 2000, an immunoglobulin product. Both of these would help protect his gut from the antibiotics.

As the months passed, Dan's Alzheimer's was stopped in its tracks. Dan said he actually felt that his short-term memory improved, though Rebecca was more cautious. "Maybe," she said in one follow-up visit, "but it's not obvious." She did agree it had stopped getting worse—and for Dan and Rebecca, a couple that had been on the brink of despair, that was a lot. They'd been on the edge of a cliff, but now they no longer lived in fear of an imminent mental drop-off.

Five years have passed since Dan's first visits, and I now see him once every three months or so. On paper, Dan isn't dramatically different from when I met him. But he's no longer in free fall. He and Rebecca have both taken big breaths and seen that he's no longer knocking at death's door. He has hope. His steep decline is over, and he still has the same job he had back then—in other words, he didn't get his promotion back, but he also didn't get the demotion he was at risk of before. He's interacting with his kids more, and he sees his grandkids more often. He's living life as though he's going to be around for a while. Things haven't been totally restored, but he's found a "new normal." He exercises, eats well, seeks out joy in his life, and cultivates relationships—all the things he knows he needs to do to maintain his current level of wellness, and possibly improve in the future.

Functional medicine isn't about making miracles. If you meet someone who says they can completely cure Alzheimer's, you're probably hearing a tall tale. But stabilizing somebody with Alzheimer's, as we did with Dan, is possible—and that's miracle enough for me.

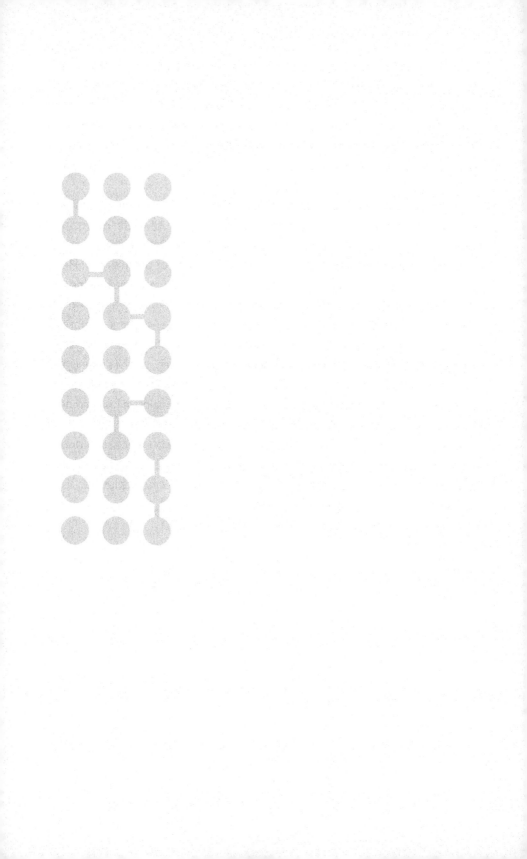

# BIOTRANSFORMATION AND ELIMINATION

**Biotransformation and Elimination** (toxicity, detoxification)

Whereas assimilation is the physiological system that deals with bringing things into the body and making them usable, biotransformation and elimination is the system that processes and excretes metabolites from the body. In addition to eliminating metabolic and digestive wastes, this system also chemically modifies substrates, including drugs and toxins (biotransforms them), to facilitate their activation and/or removal from the body.

When this system is functioning optimally, waste products from digestion and metabolism are expeditiously removed from the body via the GI tract, urinary tract, and skin; and toxins (both endogenous and exogenous) are bio-transformed and eliminated efficiently. However, many factors can impact the ability of these processes to function optimally, including increased toxic exposure, nutrient insufficiencies, metabolic dysfunction, drug interactions, and intestinal dysbiosis.[2]

At a farm pond just southwest of the Twin Cities, a group of children and parents on a nature hike noticed an abundance of odd-looking frogs. They picked up frog after frog from the pond and found that dozens were misshapen. Some were missing legs, others had extra legs, and still others had strangely shaped approximations of legs growing from their bodies. Alarmed, the parents alerted the Minnesota Pollution Control Agency in St. Paul.

It was 1995, and the story of the deformed frogs grabbed national headlines. Shortly afterwards, similar outbreaks were reported in other sites in Minnesota, Wisconsin, and even Quebec. Nearly two decades later, the mystery hasn't been definitively solved, but in the investigation, federal officials found that frog embryos raised in tap water from homes near the pond where the original discovery was made exhibited similar deformities. When the water was run through a charcoal filter, though, the abnormalities disappeared. Families consuming Minnesota water were understandably unnerved.

Many scientists regard frogs as a "sentinel species"—in other words, their general well-being serves as a harbinger of the overall health of their environment, much like the canaries whose deaths signaled to coalminers that a particular shaft wasn't safe for humans. Because they live in both land and water, and because their easily permeable skin takes in liquid from all around them, frogs may be particularly sensitive to chemical pollution in their ecosystem.

But of course, these toxins—an unavoidable reality of modern life—take their toll on all of us. Fortunately, the body has a complex and effective mechanism for ridding itself of the toxins absorbed through food, drinks, and our skin. Whereas assimilation is the physiological system that deals with bringing substances into the body and making them useable, *biotransformation and elimination* is the system that eliminates metabolic and digestive waste and chemically modifies drugs and toxins—biotransforms them—to facilitate the removal from the body.

This system, however, is finite, and many factors can impair it, including increased toxic exposure, nutrient insufficiencies, metabolic dysfunction, drug interactions, and intestinal dysbiosis, not to mention genetic factors. When that happens, our detox process can go haywire.

One significant way detoxification can go wrong is something we talked about in the previous chapter: an imbalance between phase one detoxification and phase two detoxification. When you have a toxic river flowing into your body, phase one starts churning. The toxin goes to the liver, is oxidized, and is turned into a free radical—a highly reactive chemical. But phase two—which incorporates a glucose, sulfur, or amino acid molecule and makes the free radical compound water-soluble and excretable—is highly dependent on nutrients. So, when you're nutritionally depleted and flooded with toxins, you slowly become deficient in phase two detoxification, leaving the mechanism imbalanced and your body with a backlog of free radicals.

These free radicals, hungry for electrons, tear material out of the tissue in whatever part of the body they happen to be. If the free radicals are near your coronary artery, they're going to push you toward heart disease. If they're in your brain, they may result in or accelerate neurological disease. If they're in your DNA, they could lead to cancer or other DNA damage. This damage is on a molecular level—one free radical isn't a big deal . . . but hundreds of millions, billions, or trillions of them is. And for perspective, consider this: a single puff from a cigarette contains hundreds of trillions of free radicals.

●-●-●

"If I don't get this under control, doc, I'm gonna lose my job, no question."

Rick, fifty-three, was a commercial airline pilot, and he looked the part of his glamorous profession—tall, broad shoulders, a head of salt-and-pepper hair, and an air of cool competence. But, under his confidence, he was gravely concerned about his blood pressure.

"It's high," Rick told me in the exam room. "Really high. Two-ten over one-thirty. That's way over what the FAA allows—one fifty-five over ninety-five. And I've done everything. I hate to sound desperate, but you're my last hope."

He spoke calmly, with a gregarious smile, but I knew this was serious. Flying planes had always been Rick's passion, but his hypertension was threatening to rip him away from it. He'd driven over two hours from Minneapolis, all the way to this tiny cornfield town, to see me.

I pulled out a blank timeline sheet. "Well, let's see what we can do," I said. "Tell me—when was the last time you felt truly well?"

Rick answered right away. "I felt fine until my mid-forties, but then my blood pressure started creeping up. I didn't feel immediately bad, but that was the beginning of it."

"And what happened after that?"

"Just kept going up, slowly but surely, until it hit the FAA limit a few years ago. That's when I started getting grief about it. And I'm a healthy guy. I eat plenty of fruits and vegetables. I run. And that's pretty rare for guys like me. Most pilots are living the hurry-up-and-wait lifestyle, grabbing McDonald's between flights. Not me. After the pressure started going up, I ate even better, brought all my meals from home. I find places to run in every city I stay overnight in, whether it's around the hotel or in a fitness center."

"And none of that has helped at all?"

"Nope. Seemed to make it worse, actually. So I went to my doctor, but he couldn't do anything. And he's a good guy, I trust him."

"And I see that you've even been to the Mayo Clinic—how was that?" I asked.

"It was fine, but they couldn't help, either—even though I was in the hypertension clinic! They did an angiogram and looked at my kidneys; that wasn't the problem, so they did a whole workup. Now I'm on five medications, all at moderate doses, but my blood pressure is still up, and I don't like the side effects. Some of the sexual stuff is really frustrating, and it's going to start affecting my marriage pretty soon here." Unlike a lot of my patients, Rick knew the outline of his condition and was forthcoming with details. He was laser-focused on the problem and ready to solve it.

"All right," I said, "what's your family history like? Anyone with hypertension?"

"Yep. Both my parents and two uncles on my dad's side. My dad and one uncle eventually developed heart disease. That was the basic conclusion of the Mayo people—that I was just unfortunate enough to have gotten the high-blood-pressure gene. But that can't just be *it,* can it?" Rick's straight brows gathered over his nose, his mouth tightening at the thought that there was no solution to his struggle.

"I know that sounds like a plausible story," I said, "but I don't know that it has a basis in reality. There certainly are genes associated with hypertension, but there isn't a hypertension gene.[4] So let's look around a bit and see if we can figure it out."

Rick took a deep breath and then let it out in a sigh, nodding. "Whatever we've gotta do."

Next, we delved into Rick's environmental inputs, beyond his diet, which he'd said was good. There was nothing significant—no bright red flags. But he did tell me that he had flown piston airplanes in his early days as a pilot, like most everyone starting out in aviation. Those planes—especially in the days that Rick was flying them—burned huge amounts of leaded gas. Now, most pilots do preflight walks around the plane; maybe before your last flight you saw the pilot out on the blacktop kicking the tires of the jumbo jet. For smaller planes, the pilot also has to drain the fuel sumps to make sure no water has collected there, and it's almost impossible to do that without getting gas on your hands. This meant that through Rick's contact with the fuel and fumes, he'd had an exposure to lead, although it wasn't a massive or obviously toxic one.

---

4    In fact, there are twenty-nine genetic variations across twenty-eight areas of the genome that influence blood pressure. All of these variations are in turn influenced by diet and lifestyle (http://healthland.time.com/2011/09/12/high-blood-pressure-genes-identified/).

He also told me that he frequently shot handguns, visiting indoor shooting ranges during winter and at times shooting over five hundred rounds a week. Since he was a kid, he had been loading his own ammo, a task that often left him with fingers that were grayed from the lead bullets. Despite this contact with aviation fuel and gun ammunition, his lead exposure was nothing on the order of another of my patients, who grew up in a home that doubled as an automobile body repair shop.

Nevertheless, the possibility of lead exposure got my attention. Several studies published in reputable journals have found that heart disease and hypertension have been associated with lead—and that lead is, in fact, more predictive of heart disease than cholesterol. Even though Rick's possible exposure had taken place decades before, it was entirely possible that he'd picked up more lead or other toxic metals from his surroundings and that this was the key to alleviating his high blood pressure.

●-●-●

Of course, plenty of people have exposures like Rick's but don't develop hypertension. And not all people in communities exposed to toxic waste develop illnesses. Not even all the frogs in the contaminated Minnesota pond were deformed.

This is because many people, including a good portion of my patients, have polymorphisms—common genetic mutations that cause the extreme diversity in people's ability to detoxify. These polymorphisms account for why some people can live in the most polluted place on earth and still live a healthy life, but others could live in a pristine mountain meadow with a mask and still be sick. As it turns out, there is about a 10,000 percent difference between the least efficient polymorphism and the most efficient polymorphism, in terms of the person's ability to detoxify a given pollutant.

Nevertheless, at some point, regardless of your ability to detoxify, toxins will start to impact your physiology. Many people with chronic unwellness, whether it's hypertension, chronic fatigue, or arthritis, have slowly accumulated toxins that their bodies haven't been able to eliminate. For many of my patients, the problem is chronic low-level exposure—the type we all have—combined with impaired detox capability. Sometimes the exposure can be from sources as innocuous as perfume and medications.

There was a study done for two decades in which researchers biopsied a group's fat tissue and analyzed it for pollutants. Turns out that 100 percent of people were testing positive for xylene and a host of other pollutants. Eventually, they just stopped doing the study—why keep testing if everybody has these things?

The number of pollutants we create and release into the environment is growing exponentially, and we consider many things safe even though we have minuscule data on them—certainly not the amount required to declare them harmless. Just look at plastic. When I was a kid, plastic was brittle; you could flex a cheap plastic toy and it would crack. But now we fill plastics with plasticizers to make them pliable like rubber. What most people don't realize is that these plasticizers are endocrine disrupters that interfere with human health. For example, a recent article in the *Journal of the American Medical Association* associated high levels of bisphenol A (a chemical compound used to make plastics) in the urine of children with obesity!

The dangers of such exposures are woefully understated. Researchers will do tests on new pollutants to figure out how toxic they are, but when they arrive at the permissible level, the results are seen in isolation; these researchers do not consider how that toxin might interact with detox pathways or be synergetic with other toxins. Thus, the permissible level they set is often far too high. Nevertheless, you'll hear things like, "Oh, it's perfectly safe."

Take lead, for example. In 1960, it was thought that 60 micrograms of lead per deciliter of blood was perfectly safe in children. But in 1975, they did a little more research and said, "Well, actually it looks like they should only have thirty micrograms of lead per deciliter in the blood." Any more than that, officials said, and you'd probably have a problem. Then, in 1985 they said, "Well, gee, anything more than twenty-five micrograms of lead might be dangerous." In 1991, a new study: no more than 10 micrograms of lead in a child's blood is safe. At the time, many in the complementary alternative medicine (CAM) community were seeing reports of even greater toxicity. But the establishment held fast, advising that anyone who said that 10 micrograms of lead was unsafe was a quack. But in 2012, they dropped the number again—to five micrograms per deciliter of blood.

These numbers aren't just abstractions; they have very real effects on humans. Studies of infants and children have shown that the first ten micrograms of lead per deciliter of blood may decrease the child's IQ by 7.4 points, and for every additional 10 micrograms, the child's IQ can fall by up to 4.6 points.

So, in 1960, if your child was allowed to maintain 60 micrograms per deciliter, that represented a potential thirty-point IQ loss. (I don't know about you, but I don't have 30 extra IQ points lying around.)

And that's lead by itself. What if there's also a bit of mercury, or arsenic, or PCB? There is this huge synergy between toxins that has only rarely been studied, and we don't even have a beginning of an understanding of how big the problem is. There are all kinds of pollutants in our environment, and we look at them in isolation. But whether it's deformed frogs or alarming cancer rates in humans, the problem appears to be not one main toxin but the constellation of toxicity working in concert.

Mercury and lead, already toxic on their own, become even worse when combined. In one study, small doses of mercury salt and lead salt were administered to a group of rats. Though the doses were given in amounts that would have virtually no response on their own, when combined, the salts killed every single rat in the study.[5] Just imagine what similar types of negative synergy are at work in the combinations of toxins we humans are exposed to on a daily basis.

And once pollutants are released, they don't just evaporate after a few years. DDT (dichloro-diphenyl-trichloroethane, a pesticide), which hasn't been manufactured in the United States since the 1980s, is still hanging around in the fat of polar bears and penguins. Sandra Steingraber's *Living Downstream* is a portrait of the consequences of this lingering toxicity. Steingraber, diagnosed with bladder cancer at twenty, starts out the book by discussing her mother's cancer and her grandfather's cancer. But then she slowly reveals that she actually doesn't have a family history of cancer—she was adopted. The common thread was the community her family lived in, one flooded by nasty chemicals. Study after study backs up Steingraber's thesis: that these toxins have a devastating impact on human health.

The body's finite ability to deal with these toxins—specifically, its ongoing fight to carry out phase two detoxification—sets the stage for this massive multisystem failure. Think of the detox pathways as funnels. If you're pouring one toxic substance—here represented by a glass of water—through the funnel, it will pass through without a problem. But if you're trying to pour ten

---

5    J. Schubert, E. J. Riley, S. A. Tyler, "Combined Effects in Toxicology—A Rapid Systematic Testing Procedure: Cadmium, Mercury, and Lead."

glasses of water through the same small funnel, it's going to start backing up and overflowing. Like that funnel, our detox pathways have a finite capacity to detoxify, and when we're trying to handle several synergistic toxicities at once, we run into trouble.

When you're getting more and more toxic, nutrient absorption is poor, your gut tends to get leaky, and this causes even more toxic flooding in the liver. Your liver then struggles to detoxify all of the toxic chemicals, food allergies, antigens, microbial antigens, and immune complexes, and these highly reactive toxins start leaking into the systemic circulation. Your adrenal glands, which make cortisol to help manage these inflammatory burdens, start to up-regulate (to adapt to the toxic burden by producing more countermeasures) but eventually they get tired, too—a condition we call "adrenal fatigue." When that happens, and when the situation is worsened by factors such as medication, alcohol, poor diet, and stress, your body's problem gets bigger even as its capacity to fix it becomes smaller.

●-●-●

On the day of Rick's first visit, I talked with him a bit more about his lifestyle and history, but nothing jumped out to me as a clear contributor to his persistent hypertension. So, I decided to do a few tests on him and see if the lead theory held any weight. The first test was the NutrEval—the nutritional efficiency test that I do—but I also did a provoked-urine toxic mineral analysis, where I gave him a medicine designed to pull metals out of his tissues and dump them into his urine. That would allow me to see what came out.

When I got Rick's tests back a few days later, it turned out he had really high lead and borderline high mercury. I'd developed a theory as to why this was. I have many patients who have polymorphisms in something called the metallothionein pathway, which is the pathway most involved in the detoxification of heavy metals. Let's say you or I, with our normal metallothionein pathways, can detoxify twenty-five mercury molecules per day. (I'm just making up that number for our example.) Through our environment, mainly through the fish we eat, say we take in about twenty mercury molecules every day and can successfully detoxify them. But if someone has a problem with the metallothionein pathway, perhaps they can only get rid of fifteen mercury molecules a day but are getting the same twenty we get. That means they are net positive five mercury molecules every day, and that slowly accumulates over time until, at some point, this person has enough mercury to disrupt his enzymes and he becomes symptomatic.

Since there was hypertension on both sides of Rick's family and his dad in particular, I guessed that it could well be because they all carry a polymorphism that causes the metallothionein system to be inefficient. In his test results, I found a clue that supported this theory: Rick had high copper and low zinc, which is precisely what people with this metallothionein problem typically have.

Now that I had Rick's test results and a working hypothesis as to why his hypertension wouldn't go away, I could fully fill out his matrix and present him with his story.

On his second visit, Rick was his outgoing, confident self, and was eager to hear what I had to say.

"Lay it on me, doc," he said. "I'm ready."

"Well, you don't have any significant environmental exposures that would cause this, but I believe your body is having trouble handling lead." I explained the metallothionein pathway and how his results indicated that he might carry a polymorphism that inhibited its work. "Because you have this inefficient metallothionein pathway, you've just slowly accumulated these metals. It took thirty to thirty-five years, but now you're starting to show clear signs of toxicity, the most apparent being your high blood pressure that the medicines just can't touch. I also think you're flooded with free radicals caused by your overwhelmed detox systems and the metals themselves," I added. "These are causing oxidative stress, which is closely linked to hypertension.

"Your NutrEval also showed that you're deficient in glutathione—that's a sort of super antioxidant your body makes. It's also used as a detoxification pathway, and so it may be low because it's trying to compensate for the problem with the metallothionein pathway. The results also show elevated lipid peroxides, which is oxidized fat. Oxidized metal is rusty metal; oxidized fat is rusty fat. Anyway, this is all more evidence that you're under tremendous oxidative stress, probably caused from the heavy metals."

Rick took everything in, nodding. "Not anything I could have guessed, but all makes sense," he said. "What do we do about it?"

"Well, I'd like to go ahead and start trying to detoxify your system. I'm not going to lie—it's going to be a long process. Fortunately, you won't have to change your work habits. It's not like you work at a lead–acid battery factory or anything. But it will take some work and patience."

"I'm ready, doc," Rick said. "Where do we start?"

The first phase of Rick's detoxification was a three-month nutritional fortification program. That seems like a long time, but if you really want to change the nutritional status of the cells, you need to give them time to incorporate these nutrients—just think about the fact that a red blood cell lives about 120 days. Different tissues in the body have different turnover times, and it takes as least as long as the lifespan of a red blood cell to fully incorporate a nutrient. It's not as if you can just take a vitamin, saturate your blood in a few days, and have your body rebuilt and repaired.

We put Rick on an anti-inflammatory medical food and switched him to organic foods. The switch to organic was especially important for Rick, because organic foods tend to be lower in heavy metals. Ash from municipal incinerators is often used as a mineral source in commercial fertilizer, and that's one of the main ways heavy metals get into our food. Getting him on organic-only would decrease that exposure.

Nutrition can certainly improve the body's ability to biotransform and detoxify, but I made a clear distinction to Rick: the "Nutrient of the Month" club doesn't work. You know what I mean—the nutrition and natural treatment newsletters you get that tout some different miracle food every month. They'll tell you it's the greatest thing in the world and you should eat boatloads of it, as if this one item—often some tropical fruit no one's heard of—is the ultimate cure for human illness. Then, the next month, they're on to something new.

As part of this first three-month phase, we also got Rick on several nutrients. We started him on cracked-cell chlorella, which has been shown to help detoxify heavy metals, and gave him a bunch of nutrients designed specifically to optimize detoxification and his gut function. We also gave him a complement of B vitamins and minerals and a complement of phytonutrients to help phase one and phase two detoxification. Finally, we gave him a whole set of antioxidants that work together, plus nutrients that help his body make glutathione—that super-antioxidant made inside the body.

It was important that we give Rick a full array of nutrients in this phase, because giving him just one—even a beneficial one—could actually worsen the problem. Let's say we do a nutritional efficiency test and find that a person is inefficient in using B12. So we give him more B12, and he becomes a little bit more efficient but not dramatically so. So we give him a ton more B12, and he gets even less efficient. Then we double the already-high B12 dose and he gets no better. It's because we've saturated his system with B12, and unfortunately, he's as efficient at using B12 as he's ever going to be unless the gene changes—and altering genes is something we can't do just yet.

So, when it comes to nutrition, it's not just "more is better." Instead, each of us has an optimal saturation of nutrients, and once we reach the optimal saturation, consuming more may actually have adverse consequences. Antioxidants work in what we call "redox chains," and oversupplying one link in the chain at the expense of others can actually pump up the rate of free-radical production. In one study, high doses of beta-carotene actually appeared to increase smokers' risk of getting lung cancer.[6]

During those first three months of focused nutrition, Rick did well. As we pumped him with nutrients, he stayed on his regular five medications and retained his optimism and commitment. Most important of all, he stayed patient even though his blood pressure wasn't budging much.

After three months, it was time for the next phase: treatment with oral doses of dimercaptosuccinic acid (DMSA), a chelating agent that would help get lead out of his system. DMSA mobilizes the toxins, but we had to be careful not to mobilize in excess of Rick's ability to excrete and get rid of them. Although we had hopefully banished many toxins during his three-month nutritional tune up, if the DMSA mobilized too many, we could redistribute these toxins to more sensitive organs—taking them out of the fat and sending them into the brain, for instance—and this could makes Rick sicker. To prevent this, we started him out on a small dose of DMSA. I explained that we had to do this phase slowly, because if we presented his kidney with too many toxins all at once, he wouldn't be able to excrete them all, and they'd simply be redistributed to other tissues and make him sicker.

After three months on the DMSA, we did another toxic elements test. This one showed that the lead and mercury in Rick's urine was actually *higher* than the baseline tests. When I told Rick, he looked worried, but I quickly assured him that this was actually a good sign. "Remember, this is stuff in your urine—that means we're pulling more *out* of your body."

---

6  "The Effect of Vitamin E and Beta Carotene on the Incidence of Lung Cancer and Other Cancers in Male Smokers," *The New England Journal of Medicine* (1994), accessed August 7, 2013. www.nejm.org/doi/full/10.1056/NEJM199404143301501.

At six months, Rick's lead and mercury numbers were higher yet, but he'd finally had his first breakthrough in lowering his blood pressure; it had come down about ten points on both sides—top and bottom, or systolic and diastolic. It was now about two hundred over one-twenty, which is still way too high, but it was coming down. This treatment was the first thing that had brought his blood pressure down at all. The look of relief on Rick's face at that visit was priceless.

After three more months, the amounts of lead and mercury in Rick's urine were starting to decrease—not as low as the original detoxification panel but lower than the previous one, which had been the peak. That was a good sign: it told me we were over the hump and had gotten a significant amount of the toxicity out of his system. Even more encouraging was the fact that his blood pressure had now come down another ten points on both sides.

Three months later, after a year of detoxification, his blood pressure was at one-sixty over ninety. At eighteen months: one-twenty over seventy—well under the FAA requirement. At that point, we started withdrawing one blood pressure drug every three months but continuing the DMSA. At the end of that additional fifteen months, Rick was off all his drugs and boasting a healthy blood pressure of one-twenty over seventy.

In the end, Rick's detoxification process took two and a half years. It definitely wasn't some rapid ten-day detox program. The truth is that in the majority of cases, getting to wellness takes a significant amount of time, especially when we're correcting a problem that developed over half a century of toxic exposure.

Regardless of the wait, Rick was thrilled by the results. He had understood his story and that it was going to take time and effort to recover, and he was motivated to get through it. The reward waiting on the other side was the ability to continue living his passion of flying planes—and a biotransformation and detoxification system that was back to running like the high-tech jets he flies.

# Chapter 8

# TRANSPORT

**Transport** (cardiovascular, lymphatic system)

Transport involves the movement of cargo. In the body, this includes the movement of molecules within cells, between cells and tissues, and throughout the body. Intracellular transport occurs mostly via diffusion or microtubule highways, while intercellular transport occurs in the extracellular fluids, mainly the blood, lymph, cerebrospinal fluid, and interstitial fluid.

Problems with the transport system, including the structural integrity specific to transport processes (e.g., subcellular endoplasmic reticulum, endothelial vascular functions, GI physiology, etc.) can cause dysfunction. Just as blocked highways can cripple a city, when materials cannot be transported efficiently within the body, metabolism slows and dysfunction results. Heart failure, hypertension, kidney disease, and glaucoma are all examples of dysfunction in the transport system.[2]

No matter what we happen to be doing at any given moment, our bodies are in constant motion—at least internally. Every second of the day, a complex set of processes moves cargo from where it is in the body to where it needs to be, whether it's neurotransmitters moving down the axon of a nerve cell or the blood coursing through your arteries and veins. Those processes make up the fifth area of the matrix—transport, which encompasses the movement of molecules within cells, between cells, and throughout the body.

The body's transport systems are crucial to our survival, but our understanding of why they sometimes malfunction is constantly evolving. Back in the 1970s, when I was working as a paramedic, there was a guy in the cardiac rehab center who designed special T-shirts for some of our patients. The shirts had a bright red, anatomically correct heart printed right over the spot on the chest where the wearer's real heart beats. This guy, however, had infused the shirts with some creativity; he'd depicted the human heart as a piece of plumbing, complete with sink pipes and screw-on fixtures to represent the bypassed arteries. The representation was in line with how we thought about the cardiovascular system in those days: it was a complex piece of plumbing, and if you had buildup in a pipe (the artery), you just had to unblock it like you would a hair clog with Drano.

Today, however, our understanding of cardiovascular disease has evolved. Certainly the problem—clogged arteries—is the same, as are its treatments. But we've come to see such clogging as the end result, not the problem. If you're having a heart attack, it's not because the mechanisms of transporting your blood went haywire; it's because you had other metabolic reactions that resulted in plugging of the artery. Likewise, if you have a persistent issue with circulation, it's because your heart is pumping ineffectively; you likely have inflammation of the heart (myocarditis) or an enlarged or weakened heart (myocardopathy), not some fundamental problem with transport mechanisms.

In this way, transport is different from the other areas we've talked about so far. All the nodes of the matrix are deeply intertwined—and certainly not independent functions—but when it comes to transport, the interrelation with other areas of the matrix is particularly pronounced: if you have a problem with transport, it has almost always originated in another part of the matrix. In fact, the entire matrix is like a hologram. If you have a piece of holographic film and you project through it, you get a three-dimensional representation. But you can cut a small piece of that film out and project through it and get the exact same whole picture. Similarly, each piece of the matrix contains a picture of the whole system—and nowhere is this more apparent than in transport.

Nevertheless, the function of moving things around the body is an integral part of being alive—so much so that it's still helpful to discuss transport separately. That discussion helps us better understand certain diseases—and reveals how problems in other matrix areas can rear their troublesome heads in transport-related ways.

⬤-⬤-⬤

The first few minutes of my initial chat with Jessica were a bit jarring. At a vibrant thirty-two (she could've passed for early twenties), she was at her wits' end with painful swelling of the legs and feet—what physicians call "edema." In other words, Jessica was a young woman with an old person's problem.

"I have three boys," she said. "Justin, Rich, and Chad—and after every pregnancy the swelling just got worse."

"And how old are they now?"

"Chad's my youngest. He's five now—though I can't quite believe it," she said, smiling. "They're all just over a year apart."

"So sounds like you've been dealing with this for about seven years now right?"

Jessica rolled her eyes dramatically. "Oh my god, yes. It's so awful. Do you have any idea how much I miss wearing shoes? My feet get so swollen, I pretty much live in flip-flops. And it's not so bad today, but it can turn this horrible color." She lifted her loose pant leg and showed me the outside of her shin. It was indeed dusky looking, a freckly reddish brown against her fair skin. And Jessica was a fit woman—she looked like the athletic type from the knees up. But below, the skin was bloated, ballooning around her sandals.

"And your doctor said it was . . ."

"Dermatitis," Jessica said. "That's all he said. Until I went home and Googled it, I wasn't entirely sure what that even meant. He gave me some cream for it, but after two months, nothing changed."

"Dermatitis" is a general term that refers to inflammation of the skin, often eczema. It was a pretty run-of-the-mill diagnosis for someone like her, who'd been suffering from swelling in the same area for over seven years.

"And, I mean, what you're seeing now—that's *nothing*," she said. "Compared to how it swelled up after I had Justin? Oh my god, nothing. After that delivery, both legs swelled up to four inches bigger than before. I looked like the elephant man. With Rich and Chad, it was bad, but not that bad. And after Chad, it got maybe half better. It's stayed that way for five years now."

"I'd imagine this affects you on a day-to-day level, right? Why don't you tell me about that?"

"Well, first of all, it's really embarrassing." Jessica looked down at her feet. Her toes were painted a cheerful coral color, as though to distract from the inflammation. "I never wear shorts or skirts anymore, even in summer. But I guess more importantly, it's just the pain, this deep ache. The only way to make it better is to kick my legs up for a while. But with three kids and a full-time job . . . it's tough to find the time. Lots of days I just push through it."

"Do you mind if I take a look?" I asked. I was sure there was more behind this severe swelling than a simple case of dermatitis. And it was going to take more than a prescription for cortisone cream to get her some relief and find the underlying cause of the edema.

Jessica shook her head and again lifted the hem of her pants. Leaning forward, I pressed a finger to the skin of her shin. It puffed out around my finger like a pillow, and when I pulled away, my finger left a dent that would stay on her leg for nearly thirty minutes. She had all the classic symptoms of a condition called venous stasis, where blood collects and stagnates in the legs.

"Well, Jessica," I said, "I don't think this is as simple as a skin condition. I think a problem with your veins is causing all this."

"My veins?" Jessica asked, instinctively glancing down at her legs as though she might be able to see the veins through her pants and the problem in them beyond that. "But isn't that . . . I mean, I'm only thirty-two. That can't be normal."

Jessica was absolutely right. Why was she, decades younger than the typical edema sufferer, dealing with this? What was going on here?

●-●-●

Whatever was happening in Jessica's body had manifested itself in the transport area of the functional medicine matrix. When transport happens within cells, it's typically through the vast network of mocrotubules within every cell. These structures, which make up what is called the cytoskeleton, are essentially super highways for motor proteins, molecular motors that carry cargo around the cell.

Transport between cells happens through fluids like blood, lymph, and cerebrospinal fluid. Indeed, one of the most important functions of transport is keeping the cardiovascular system running, and this was where Jessica's body seemed to be running into trouble. Let's zoom in for a moment on how the body moves blood around—that will help us get a close-up view of how transport works . . . and discover the root of Jessica's edema.

When you inhale, you draw in air from your environment. That air can be crisp and oxygen-rich if you're standing, say, in a mountain meadow, or it can be filthy and toxin-filled, as when you're pulling it in through the butt of a Marlboro. The air then travels down the windpipe, or trachea, into one of the two bronchi that branch off into the lungs. There, air is pushed to the alveoli—Latin for "little cavities"—where it finally makes contact with the bloodstream. The gasses in the air diffuse across the pulmonary membrane and attach to hemoglobin molecules inside the red blood cells rushing by. Each freshly loaded red blood cell is then off to the left atrium of the heart. From there, it's pumped through a valve into the left ventricle and then pushed out into the body.

The blood now goes through the largest artery in your body, the aorta, which comes out of the top of your heart, makes a large sweeping turn, and then heads down your chest and abdomen and heads for your feet. Along its course, there are branches that go to your right arm, up to your neck, down your left arm, down into your abdomen and other organs, and then finally your legs.

As the blood moves away from the heart and toward the extremities, though, the pressure behind it drops; the arteries branch into smaller arteries that branch into still tinier arteries that branch into arterials that branch into arterial capillaries that branch into capillaries that branch into venous capillaries. By the time blood is in the toes, it still needs the pressure to get back through the vein system and to the heart and lungs for re-oxygenation. The leg muscles, along with the valves in the veins of the leg, are what pump the blood back upward.

When the leg muscles and vein valves don't effectively force the blood back toward the heart, the old static blood swishes around in your legs, which causes swelling, skin discoloration, and even clots (thrombosis). Sure enough, as I talked to Jessica further, she revealed she had had a blood clot in her right leg after one of her pregnancies. It had since cleared up, but it was another clue that venous stasis—this pooling of blood in the veins—was Jessica's problem.

Her veins, I suspected, weren't effectively pumping nutrients back to her heart. Those brown, dusky areas on her legs were caused because the stagnant, less oxygenated blood was just sitting there (hence the "stasis" part of venous stasis); that skin was being malnourished.

The question to answer was this: why wasn't Jessica's transport system succeeding in moving her blood around efficiently? Like the other processes we've talked about so far, the transport system is a chain; any breakdown along the way could be leading to the problem.

Weakness of the leg muscles, or of the valves inside veins, is one significant factor in venous stasis and in clot formation. Effective circulation in the far-away reaches of the body is dependent on healthy muscles and healthy valves inside the veins. Every time you flex your calf or thigh muscle, you squeeze the soft walls of the veins, causing blood to squirt back to the heart, while the valves make sure the blood keeps flowing in the right direction.

Our bodies are whole systems designed to be moving around—a lot—and this motion helps the veins keep blood moving back up to the heart, against gravity. In our need for frequent movement, we are a little like sharks, which pull oxygen out of the water by swimming through it; the water flows into their mouths and out the gills. But if a shark stops swimming, it drowns. The constant movement is so important that sharks only sleep in half their brain at a time.

We, too, need to keep moving to circulate our blood back to our heart efficiently. In our highly sedentary society, that becomes a big problem. Even if you're not sitting at a desk all day, sitting on a cramped flight for as little as three hours can be a problem, especially when you're stuck with your knees crammed against the seat in front of you, your chair upright, and your table in the locked position, with the two big guys on either side of you stealing your armrests. Because you're hardly using your muscles at all in situations like this, the blood tends to pool in the veins.

Another cause of edema can be toxins of almost any kind. How do toxins cause vein problems? By interfering with the integrity of the capillary beds—networks of capillaries that support a particular organ. These capillary beds constantly allow themselves to leak fluid in and then close to expel it; that's how you get exchange of the fluid that flows between cells. But toxins can cause capillary beds to open but not re-close, causing the fluid of the blood to leak out and become swelling in the peripheral areas.

As I went over Jessica's symptoms in more detail, she mentioned that they worsened right before her period. This didn't surprise me—swelling is, of course, a common symptom of PMS. During the week before a woman's period, the hormone milieu changes, and—like toxins—these hormones can cause capillaries to become leaky. For most women, the resultant edema is trivial, but for some it can become significant: they can't fit into their shoes, they get pain in their feet, or their skin turns purple—all because the transport blockage has caused poor nutrition and poor oxygenation of the tissues.

Before Jessica's first visit ended, she also gave me another important piece for her timeline: every female on her mother's side had varicose veins—a condition closely related to what Jessica was dealing with. Varicose veins happen when a valve malfunctions and allows blood to collect in the vein; this causes the vein to become enlarged and painful. Jessica's veins weren't badly varicose, but this bit of information told me that she probably had a genetic predisposition to her transport problems.

All in all, Jessica's matrix was fairly clean by the time we finished filling it out, with pretty much everything showing up in the transport section. (This confinement to one sector is relatively unusual, but for the purposes of this book, I have chosen cases that more or less isolate a single area of the matrix.) But before I could tell Jessica exactly how we were going to address her venous stasis, I needed her to get a special type of ultrasound called a venous incompetency study.

The results came back after a few days, and Jessica was back in my office.

"Hi, Jessica," I said as I walked into the exam room. "Got some pretty good news for you. Believe it or not, the ultrasound showed that your leg circulation was fairly healthy. We've got two kinds—deep circulation and superficial circulation—and the systems are connected by what we call 'perforators.' Think of deep and superficial like the two vertical sides of a ladder; the perforators are the rungs."

"Mmhmm, right," Jessica said, prodding me along.

"So your deep circulation in the legs is perfectly healthy, and all the perforators are fine. Even the superficial is moderately healthy, but you do have one section that is what we call 'incompetent,' meaning it isn't working properly. The incompetent spot is right on the lateral part of the shin where your worst swelling and discoloration are—and the same place you told me you were pretty sure was where you had the blood clot during your last pregnancy.

"So what I think you have here is a self-perpetuating problem," I continued. "You got this really bad edema after your first pregnancy; the edema caused bad circulation; the bad circulation caused toxicity; the toxicity caused more capillary leakiness; which caused even more edema, and so on. One segment of vein started it—the incompetent place I was talking about—but then there was this deeper, more distal metabolic process that created a continuous toxic environment, and that's what's causing this ongoing leakiness. The fact that your mom's side of the family deals with varicose veins tells me that you may have been predisposed to this, too, and that could have been a factor."

From there, Jessica was eager to move on to solutions, and for the remainder of the visit, we went over a six-part varicose vein treatment protocol. I was certain it would bring some level of relief to her ailing transport system, even if it would take some patience and effort.

The first step was to **improve bowel function**. Jessica looked puzzled when I asked about this at her first appointment. I could pretty much read her mind: *What the hell do my swollen legs have to do with bowel movements?* But they are connected. As the blood tries to make its way from the feet back to the heart, the veins have to pump it through the abdomen. If you're chronically constipated, you have more stool weight on your vena cava—the major blood pipe in that area. And to make matters worse, you're frequently bearing down, which pushes blood backward, against the valves of the vein and back toward the swollen feet.

In her first visit, Jessica had glossed over this issue, insisting everything was fine, no problem. But now, perhaps feeling more comfortable, she opened up and said she did in fact have a tendency to be constipated. Voila—a new area of the matrix to address: assimilation. Before moving on, I went over the five Rs with her (see page 48), and explained that if we could fix her GI issues and constipation, she'd speed up progress on her venous stasis.

Second, I wanted Jessica to **decrease muscle strain**—especially from bearing down—as she was doing while constipated or when picking up something heavy. We talked about how to lift by squatting down rather than bending at the waist. When her kids crawled up on an ottoman or a chair, I asked her to bend at the knee to lift them up instead of just grabbing them off the floor the way she usually did. Again, the goal was to decrease the abdominal pressure that would make the veins work harder.

The third element of the protocol involves me asking the patient to **lose body weight**. Body weight, especially abdominal weight, puts external pressure on the large veins in the abdomen. When these veins are taxed in this way, they require more internal pressure to get the blood back to the heart. Fortunately, Jessica was already at a good BMI, so we didn't do anything here.

The fourth element is designed to help the veins out with some motion—I wanted Jessica to **pump her calf muscles**. Because Jessica's legs hurt so much, she'd kept off her feet as much as possible, but we put her on an easy daily walking program. I also asked her to regularly pump her calves, which she would do by lying on her back, lifting the leg, and pointing the toe toward her head, then away, holding it for a few seconds each time. We also put her in support stockings that would give external support, holding all of her muscles tight and helping push those veins back together. I asked her to wear them all day every day, the only exception being when she was sitting with her legs up in the evening.

The last way to lower vein pressure is to **undergo surgical treatment** of the veins. I hoped we wouldn't get there, so I moved quickly on, talking about things Jessica could do in upcoming months to help her veins grow healthier.

As usual, we started with diet. Jessica's eating habits didn't need an overhaul, but I did ask her to pump up her fruit and vegetable intake. We also needed to protect the veins with extra antioxidant support, so I gave her a "super green food," which is a fruit-and-vegetable powder. I had her take a scoop of the super green food twice a day; each one would have the same amount of antioxidants as about twenty servings of fruits and vegetables.

Because we know that veins need a lot of collagen, I put her on extra vitamin C and a multivitamin. Omega-3 fatty acids would also provide support for the veins, as well as three herbs thought to help venous disease: horse chestnut, ginko biloba, and gotu kola. Some studies show that horse chestnut was actually as effective in treating swelling as wearing support stockings.

Once we'd covered what her next few months would look like, I finished up by running through some of the surgical options for varicose veins and swelling. But Jessica was emphatic that she didn't want to have surgery. Her attitude was refreshing—most people want the quick fix, even if there's a potentially healthier and less risky path.

"Great," I told her as she gathered her things to go. "I don't think surgery is your best option right now either. I think you'll see good progress if you stick to all the things we've talked about—but especially the stockings. Bottom line is, as long as you can tolerate these stockings, let's keep going and see where we get."

"I can do stockings," Jessica said cheerily. "Thank god it's winter."

⬤–⬤–⬤

For the next year and a half, Jessica came back every three months, and every time she was spunky and upbeat—old lady stockings and all. "You know, my legs feel really good as long as I'm wearing these things," she said on her first follow-up visit. "Every once in a while I take them off and my legs swell again, but I don't think it's as bad as before." On each subsequent visit, Jessica said the same thing: she was swelling less and less. At eighteen months, she was ready to try losing the stockings for a while. I told her to go for it.

Jessica has now been completely out of the stockings for about a year and a half. By improving the circulation, optimizing her diet, wearing the stockings, walking frequently, and pumping her calves, she slowly but surely expelled all that extraneous fluid out of her tissues and improved the nutritional balance in them. Through supplementation, we had also managed to help the veins repair themselves to some degree.

Jessica is a pretty extreme case—most patients don't see full recovery without some kind of surgical intervention. But despite her dramatic improvement, I recommended that she stay on the horse chestnut and super green food for life. Because of her genetic predisposition, I was concerned that she could have recurrence. Does Jessica need these? We're not sure. Will she stay on them for life? Probably not. At some point she's likely to get tired of taking them, and then we'll see whether she relapses or not.

•-•-•

Some months before I met Jessica, I had another patient—Carly—who had strikingly similar problems. But Carly's story goes to show that sometimes surgery *is* necessary to fix a transport problem.

Carly was forty-three and also suffering from swollen legs and bulging veins. She'd gotten her first spider veins as a girl, after a softball smacked her on the calf. They'd bugged her all her life, and then when she became pregnant, she got a varicose vein in the same calf. A second pregnancy followed, and the varicose veins proliferated and worsened. By the time she came to me, the insides of her legs were lumpy with stiff, bloated veins.

Carly's ultrasound was quite different from Jessica's: Carly had gross incompetence of her entire great saphenous veins, the largest superficial vein in the leg, compared to Jessica's one small abnormal segment. Despite the greater damage, we tried the conservative approach, putting Carly on supplements and giving her the stockings.

But within months, Carly was back and needing a new approach. The stockings had become the bane of her existence, and they weren't even helping that much. Based on her lack of progress, it became clear that the method that worked for Jessica was a day late and a dollar short when it came to Carly. She'd waited too long, and it was now clear that no amount of surgical stockings and horse chestnut would fix her.

I like to remind people that functional medicine isn't always about taking an herb; it is sometimes about doing what needs to be done physiologically to fix a problem. Functional medicine does have the power to fix conditions nutritionally, but sometimes—as it was for Carly—nutrition alone is too little, too late.

We soon had Carly scheduled for an endovenous procedure, where we slide a catheter into the incompetent segment of the vein. A local anesthetic causes the vein to become numb and squeeze down around the catheter. The catheter then heats up to 120°C and kills that segment of the vein. We then pull it back and repeat until the faulty vein is put out of commission—all through a single needle with little or no pain. It is now a procedure with nominal down time, though it wasn't always that way. The procedure's evolution has been like that of gall bladder surgery; in the old days, you would have a big scar and spend several days in the hospital. But now it's a few Band-Aids and you're home on the same day. Likewise, we're now able to kill the vein with minimal invasion.

You may think, *Huh? How are you helping things if you're killing the vein?* But the eliminated vein was incompetent anyway, because its valves were no longer working. All it was doing was swishing blood back and forth, not contributing to circulation and transport. When you take that vein out, the blood starts using the perforators as an alternate route to get to deep circulation (which, in Carly, was healthy). Then, the smaller, accessory saphenous veins branching off from the removed vein start to dilate and take over its function, thus improving overall circulation.

Carly's procedure went off without a hitch. Afterward, she wore a stocking—albeit begrudgingly—twenty-four hours a day for the first three days and then every day during the day for a month. At the end of that month, she was pleased to see that her varicose veins had dramatically improved. At the one-month mark, the swelling was gone, the pain was gone, and she was thrilled. At the three-month follow-up, all of her varicose veins were completely invisible. Even though it had taken surgery, we'd patched up her transport system, and her body was now back to moving cargo around to where it was needed, free of obstruction.

# Chapter 9

# COMMUNICATION

**Communication** (endocrine, neurotransmitters, immune messengers)

The communication system in the body encompasses all the signaling interactions that occur within and between cells. Cells are constantly in contact with their environment, sending and receiving signals with their neighbors and, in some cases, with other cells throughout the body. Optimal function in the communication system involves cells and organs sending, receiving, and responding appropriately to signals from other cells.

The communication system is broad and includes several types of signals used to communicate in the body, including hormones, neurotransmitters, cytokines, paracrine factors, and other signaling molecules. Dysfunctions in messaging processing can have major repercussions on body functions.

Examples of common dysfunctions involving failure of communication processing include depression, hypothyroidism, insulin resistance, and rheumatoid arthritis.[2]

Few women relish the thought of going through menopause. *Oh my god,* they think. *I'm going to get hot flashes and night sweats. And my memory!*

Many of these women turn to a fast-growing group of physicians who brand themselves as "anti-aging" doctors—an appealing title indeed. These physicians have a solution ready for menopausal women: hormone replacement therapy. During menopause, when a woman's ovaries cease to produce eggs, levels of two hormones—estrogen and progesterone—fall, and the anti-aging doctor's fundamental belief is that the solution is replacing them, maintaining the woman at "youthful" levels of hormones. I call these doctors the "all hormones all the time" group. In the past decade, their popularity has exploded.

The anti-aging crowd has solutions for men, too. Unlike women—who are tasked with having children and who thus possess complicated and rather miraculous hormonal machinery—men's endocrine system is more straight-forward. Nevertheless, males also undergo significant hormonal changes as they age, and many look to testosterone as a way of regaining youthful vitality.

It's quite common, nowadays, for middle-aged guys to show up in my office convinced their testosterone is dropping. "I just don't have the zest I used to," they say. "I think I have Low T. I saw that commercial on TV and it described me perfectly." Although it's natural for testosterone to fall as a man ages, a pronounced drop in it can cause problems. This lowering is called andropause (or man-opause), and it can cause loss of muscle mass, strength, energy, and ambition. Pharmaceutical companies have jumped in with solutions, selling various hormones with catchy marketing campaigns.

Sure, hormone replacement can work for people, especially in the short term. It's a quick fix that holds a lot of fascination. But a functional medicine doctor is going to take a more nuanced approach, saying, "Let's look at the entire system and understand the balance that needs to happen." We recognize **hormone-related problems**—whether it's premenstrual syndrome (PMS), menopause related, hyper- or hypothyroidism, diabetes, or a host of other difficulties—as part of the next section of the matrix we're going to discuss: *communication*.

Communication runs the gamut from subcellular signaling to cell-to-cell signaling to communicating with people and community. We're going to talk about the psychosocial aspect of communication in chapter 11, so our discussion here will explore biochemical signaling—hormones. These chemicals, produced and released by glands throughout the body, carry messages to the trillions of cells that make up our bodies.

But there's a whole other side to the hormone story that the traditional approach doesn't tell. The efficacy of hormones can be affected by chronic inflammation and by problems with the detoxification process (hormones have to be done away with eventually, and the intermediate metabolites that result from an ineffective detox process can cause symptoms that mimic those of a hormone imbalance). And—like most molecular interactions in the body—the interaction between hormones and the receptors that receive them is like that of a lock and a key; the hormone is the key and the hormone receptors the lock. Sometimes, the question isn't "Do we have enough keys floating around in the body" but "How easy is it for the key to get into the lock?" and "How well maintained and well lubricated is the lock?" This declining sensitivity of the receptor is an issue the traditional approach largely overlooks. Many men and women don't need extra hormones at all. They simply need the nutrients that will help their body maintain receptor sensitivity—in other words, help the body keep its locks tuned up so that communication and signaling happens effectively.

◆-◆-◆

"I was terrified—absolutely petrified—that I was pregnant," said Jane, the lovely forty-eight-year-old who sat in my exam room. "This was last year, and I . . . my period was just so late, and I had no signs of menopause, nothing like hot flashes or insomnia."

"How late was that period?" I asked.

"Two months! Can you imagine?" said Jane, laughing. "At my age? My youngest is fifteen now and having another one *certainly* wasn't on my agenda."

"But it turned out just to be late, right?"

"Correct. But after that is when I started noticing my body going a bit haywire."

"Before that, did you feel truly well, or have you had any other health problems?" I asked.

Jane pushed a strand of her shoulder-length white hair behind her ear as she thought for a moment. She was clearly a go-getter—very perky, though she did have dark circles under both eyes. "Yes, I would say . . . I would say that before that I was fully well. No significant health difficulties to report. Certainly nothing long-lasting."

"All right. And can you tell me a bit more about what it's been like since you missed that first period?"

"I can't say it's a riveting tale," Jane said dryly. "The periods were the first problem. Since I finally got that one, they've been irregular. Some months I don't get one at all. I'm getting multiple hot flashes on most days. It's difficult for me to sleep most nights, too. Meanwhile, my mind seems to be deteriorating at an alarming rate. The lack of sleep could be part of that, I suppose, but I went from being able to juggle thirty-nine things at once to forgetting things constantly. I left my son at karate once, I pause forever when people ask for my phone number, I'm always losing items around the house—things like that."

"Anything else?" I asked.

"Well, mainly it's feeling like an octogenarian when I'm not even fifty yet," she said. "What's it going to be like when I'm actually eighty? But there's also the irritability. It was the funniest thing how I realized I was even irritable, actually. I went to our family doctor, and as I was telling him about all this, I said, 'And gosh, I don't know what's wrong with my husband—he's such a jerk these days!' My doctor asked me a few questions about it and suddenly I realized . . . holy cow, he's turning into a jerk right before my period!" Jane laughed her infectious laugh. "Obviously, it was me, not him."

Jane's primary physician had helped her along to this realization. He did his best using the current standard of care, but his treatment of the problem hadn't been effective so far. Being a fairly traditional doctor—not part of the new "all hormones all the time" wave—he wasn't necessarily eager to put Jane on hormones, so he took the approach most physicians would: he first tried to treat her *symptoms*—rather than the causes—with medication.

This is what most people find when they show up at a doctor's office with symptoms of a hormone imbalance. For younger women, these symptoms might include PMS, polycystic ovary disease, endometriosis (a condition in which cells from the lining of the uterus grow outside the uterine cavity), or PMDD (premenstrual dysphoric disorder, a severe form of PMS). In these cases, the doctor would probably prescribe Motrin, an antidepressant, a beta-blocker, or an alpha-blocker to minimize symptoms. The same would be prescribed to older women experiencing menopausal symptoms like night sweats, hot flashes, fatigue, memory loss, and hair loss where they want it and growth where they don't. And that's exactly what Jane's doctor had done—put her on an antidepressant.

"It's not working, though," Jane explained. "I mean, I'm not depressed. Why would I be on an antidepressant? I've never been depressed! And still, this lack of energy, the moodiness, the forgetfulness, the hot flashes, all of it—it's not getting better. I can hardly lead a simple PTA meeting anymore, I'm so cranky and forgetful."

"Well," I said, "your doctor didn't put you on an antidepressant because he thinks you're depressed. He put you on it because these medications seem to be at least somewhat effective in managing the symptoms of perimenopause and menopause. Since the publication of one particular women's health study several years ago, doctors have been very reluctant to use hormones—the risks of conventional hormones now appear to outweigh the benefits." I scribbled a few final notes and said, "But don't worry. We're going to see what we can do for you."

As I was plugging Jane's recent experience with the antidepressant into her timeline, she somewhat sheepishly offered her own suggestion for how we could get her back to normal. "I've been reading about bioidentical hormone replacement," she said. "I was thinking that might be an option. I read Suzanne Somers's book and did quite a lot of online research. From what I'm reading, it seems to work wonders."

●-●-●

The "all hormones" team had struck again. Don't get me wrong—I'm sure Suzanne Somers is well intentioned. And hormone replacement *can* do some good for people who are in crisis because of a hormone imbalance.

Say a woman is having a hot flash every ten minutes all day long, and is sweating through the night and not sleeping. In that case, it's perfectly reasonable to use hormone replacement in the short term. But where functional medicine doctors and the "all hormones" crowd part is what happens next— while the latter would advise the woman to keep her hormone levels similar to those she'd had in her youth, a practitioner of functional medicine would look for a more comprehensive plan that would eventually get her off hormone replacement. (The topic of bioidentical hormone replacement therapy is *big* and would require a book this size to do it justice. Let's just say that, in general, less is more when it comes to hormones.)

Functional medicine recognizes that the body's communication system is complex and needs to be balanced, and that the fall in hormone levels as a person ages may be completely natural. In fact, as we get older and our hormone levels decline, our incidence of hormone-related cancer increases, suggesting that this decline may in fact be protective. Whatever the case, it's clear that pumping the system full of hormones can actually cause major problems.

It used to be that we thought giving hormones to women in menopause would actually help protect their heart, but it turns out that such protection, if it's there at all, is minimal. And, two common types of hormone—Premarin, estrogen in pill form, and Provera, a synthetic form of progesterone—have been shown to increase a woman's risk of both breast cancer and uterine cancer. ("Bioidentical" hormone therapy would avoid both Premarin and Provera;

the term "bioidentical" simply means the hormones used are precisely the same as those the body makes. Bioidentical hormone replacement therapy would use actual human female estrogens, while Provera is a synthetic created in a lab and Premarin is derived from the pregnant mare's urine.)

In men, too, addition of hormones to the communication system can cause unexpected problems. As men age, their biochemistry is altered, and they tend to become better at turning testosterone into estrogen. So imagine the guy who sees the "Low T" commercial goes to his doctor, gets tested, and is given extra testosterone because, sure, his levels were a little low. Well, if the root problem is that his body is converting too much testosterone into estrogen, the doctor has in effect added fuel to the fire. Testosterone will go up, but at the same time, estrogen levels will rise, too. What if we instead looked at the whole system and gave this patient nutrients that would inhibit the conversion of testosterone to estrogen? The testosterone level would elevate a little and the estrogen would go down a little—in other words, he'd get closer to a normal balance.

The delicate, interconnected nature of the endocrine system is part of why hormone replacement is so difficult. You're trying to influence this dynamic balance in the body, and it's not always clear what path is best. If a woman's estrogen is higher than her progesterone, do you raise the progesterone or lower the estrogen? The challenge is to get everything to work together in a normal physiological, age-appropriate way. (Unlike the "all hormones all the time" crowd and the "anti-aging" doctors, practitioners of functional medicine typically talk about "healthy" or "graceful" aging rather than any kind of miraculous turnaround of the process.)

Functional medicine's premise when it comes to this part of the body's communication system is that it's better to focus on receptor sensitivity and hormone detox pathways than on the raw amount of a hormone in the body—in other words, better to ensure that the locks and keys are functioning optimally before simply throwing a ton more keys in.

❖❖❖

Fortunately, Jane brought up hormone replacement as a suggestion; she wasn't dead-set on getting it. She was open-minded and analytical, so all her reading didn't preclude her from listening to my thoughts on her problem.

I first explained the lock-and-key analogy, describing how our hormone receptors can become less sensitive as we grow older and how chronic inflammation and detoxification problems play a role in the hormonal communication process. She leaned forward, nodding, hanging on every word. This was a perspective she hadn't heard before.

I also explained how her lifestyle could be contributing to the problem. "In many less industrialized countries—at least the ones that aren't war-torn—women don't experience symptoms of menopause like women in developed countries do," I said. "That may be because of stress. Every time somebody changes lanes right in front of you too fast, every time you get a letter from the IRS, every time you have a confrontation at one of your PTA meetings—you have a stress response. When we were evolving, that stress response would've been reserved for when a saber-toothed tiger jumped out in front of you, but now we have stress responses every day.

"As your ovaries start to slow down and stop making hormones, your adrenal glands partially take over, and it's a combination of the ovaries and adrenal glands that get you through menopause. So if your adrenals are already constantly stressed out with a million things in your day and your ovaries are starting to slow down at the same time, you get more significant perimenopausal symptoms.

"There's also a dietary component to it," I continued. "I know you have a pretty good diet, but eating more foods that are rich in what have traditionally been called phytoestrogens may help with some of this. I actually prefer to use the term *phytoserm* rather than *phytoestrogens*. *Phyto* refers to plants, while the *serm* stands for 'selective estrogen receptor modulator.' Thus, this term indicates that the plant-derived compounds can selectively modulate the way estrogen and the receptor interact. In a way, these compounds become what herbalists call "adaptogens"—regulators that help move the body in the direction of balance. I also prefer the term *phytoserm* because if you say 'phytoestrogens,' some women think 'Oh no, I am not supposed to take estrogens because it raises my risk of cancer.' But phytoestrogens have never been shown to do that. And in places where many of these are eaten—like in places where people eat a lot of soy—women tend to have fewer menopausal issues. There's even one language that doesn't have a word for hot flashes.

"Do you think these other ways of addressing the problem are going to work as well as hormones would?" Jane asked. "My other doctor was reluctant about using them, too, but . . . at the end of the day, I want something that works."

"Here's the thing, Jane," I said. "Hormone replacement is going to give you a quick result. You'd probably feel different in a couple of days. But I'd like to try to balance you out in a less severe way."

"I'm on board," she said after a moment of thought. "I'll do whatever you think best—as long as it helps me stop feeling like an old woman."

●–●–●

Before Jane left, I ordered two tests that would help us develop a treatment strategy. The first was a comprehensive blood test that looked not only at hormone levels—progesterone, testosterone, DHEA, estrogen—but also how those hormones are metabolized through two main detox pathways, and whether a breakdown in phase 2 detox is letting harmful reactive intermediates roam free in the body. (When the detox process breaks down and fails to dispose of these reactive intermediates, the side effects can be similar to symptoms of PMS and menopause.)

The second test was a red blood cell fatty acid analysis that would tell me Jane's fat balance and, thus, how fluid her cell membranes were. The cell membrane is a lipid bilayer—in other words, it's made up of two layers of fat. Floating around on that membrane like little islands are the receptors. If the fats you've incorporated into your membrane are stiffer fats, you're going to have stiffer membranes, which means the receptors can't float around as easily and do their job.

To get a general idea of where Jane was before the fatty acid test came in, I went back to her dietary history and focused on the types of fats she ate, asking how often she ate fats that tended to be solid at room temperature as opposed to liquid at room temperature; this is a way of asking how much saturated versus unsaturated fat she was eating. We get a lot of these solid fats in our standard American diet, and this generally contributes to the stiffness of our cell membranes. Jane, however, had a better-than-average diet; she didn't eat much junk food or trans fats, ate plenty of fruits and vegetables, and ate fish at least once a week.

It would be about two weeks before Jane's test results came in, but in the meantime, I asked her to add two things to her diet. The first was flaxseed meal, which you can find in the health food section of nearly any grocery store. I recommend that my patients like Jane work themselves up to three tablespoons a day. You can throw the flaxseeds into a coffee grinder, make them into a nice powder, and take them by the spoonful or mix it in your yogurt or salad. These flaxseeds contain lignans, which help modulate and optimize detoxification of hormones. (Flaxseeds do have a lot fiber in them, so you may want to work *slowly* up to three tablespoons to avoid gas and bloating.)

Second, I asked Jane to incorporate a serving a day of some kind of soy into her diet, whether it was soymilk or tofu. I wanted her to get those phytoserms that would help modulate how her estrogens interacted with the estrogen receptors; improving that interaction often brings things back into balance.

With those directives—flaxseed and soy—I sent Jane off for two weeks.

●-●-●

"Does this stuff make your hair nicer?" Jane asked right at the start of her next visit. Her eyes were bright, the circles beneath them lightened.

"Sometimes," I replied. "Has something changed?"

"Well, maybe it's in my head, but my hair just seems healthier. My nails, too—they don't seem to be chipping as much."

"I hear that a lot, actually," I said. "I think it has a lot to do with the healthy fats you're getting from the flaxseed."

"Whatever it is, I approve," Jane laughed.

"So you've been pretty good about getting that flaxseed and soy, then?" I asked.

"Definitely. I've been using soymilk in my cereal and eating tofu on days I skip the cereal. And I've been eating the flaxseed, too."

"Great," I said. "Has there been any change in your symptoms?"

"The hot flashes are a bit better—I don't feel like I'm about to spontaneously combust anymore. I'd say I'm waking up about half as often as before. All in all, I'm better, but I'd still say far from well."

"That's to be expected," I said. "If you'd gone the hormone replacement route, you'd likely be seeing more dramatic effects. But I still think this is the right way to go, long term."

"Well, I will tell you this—it's working better than anything I've tried so far."

We now had Jane's fatty acid test back, and it showed that her omega-3 fats—the fats we get from fish, nuts, and seeds—were in the normal range, but a little on the low end, and the same was true of her omega-9 fats (like those found in olive oil). Her omega-6 fats were normal, but they were in the high normal range, right up against the upper limit. Her saturated fats were normal, but also in the upper normal range, while her trans fats—those most dangerous to her health—were very good, quite low.

On first blush, you might think Jane's fatty acid analysis looked as it should—everything in the normal range, right? But if you look at the ratio of omega-6 fats to omega-3 and omega-9 fats, you see that the proportion is skewed: the analysis indicated a relative imbalance of omega-3 fats. She had a pro-inflammatory fatty-acid profile, and because of the relatively high saturated fats, her cell membranes were likely stiffer than ideal. I got to the bottom of it by asking more about her cooking habits. It turned out that she always used vegetable oil to cook. I told her to try switching to olive oil, which would help lower some of her omega-6s and would raise her omega-9s.

We also looked at Jane's hormone profile, which showed normal postmenopausal hormone levels. However, her hormone detoxification pathways were not quite as normal. She tended to detoxify through the 16-hydroxyestrone pathway more than the 2-hydroxyestrone pathway. This meant that she was creating active metabolites of her estrogens. It just so happens that flaxseed and soy block the 16 pathway and favor the 2 pathway. I hoped continued use of these foods in her diet would further improve her symptoms.

To help explain the rest of the changes and strategize on how to implement them, I brought in a lifestyle coach to help Jane work out planning and recipes. To help keep up those omega-3s, we asked her to keep eating fish, nuts, and seeds. She pushed back a little on the nuts and seeds; like many women, she was watching her figure, and she had heard they were fattening. But we explained that they were full of healthy fats and that we were only asking her to eat a small palm full per day (about a third of a cup).

I also wanted her to pull back on red meat. Jane had an affinity for cheeseburgers, the one spot on her otherwise excellent diet, but the beef contained more omega-6s (and specifically arachidonic acid, a precursor to pro-inflammatory pathways in the body), and we wanted to keep those down.

We also gave Jane a strong fish oil supplement to support the omega-3 fats; the supplement would give her about 3,000 milligrams of EPA and DHA (the "active ingredients" in fish oil) every day, whereas most people typically get a few hundred milligrams daily. This boost of fish oil would also reduce inflammation in her body, which was yet another distraction from proper functioning of her hormone receptors. The EPA component would not only increase the anti-inflammatory precursors in her system, but also block the arachidonic acid from entering the inflammatory pathways.

Finally, because she'd experienced a partial response to the soy and the flaxseed, I added one more supplement—this one made with kudzu, the invasive Asian vine that is taking over the south but is a great source of phytoserms. Like soy and flaxseed, kudzu would help her favor the 2-hydroxyestrone pathway for detoxification, reducing the active metabolites in her system and thus the pressure on her body's detox system.

By her second follow-up visit, Jane was virtually free of perimenopausal symptoms. She was delighted, and so was I. Her endocrine system was now operating effectively, and the hormones throughout her body were successfully communicating with their targets. And we'd done it in a short period of time, without meddling directly with her hormone levels. Jane had decided to pass up the quick-fix solution and opt for a more nuanced approach. It took a little more work on her part, but ultimately, I think she was better off for it.

All I asked Jane to do from there on out was the flax; she was free to wean herself off of all the other supplements. She did it over the next three months—all without the return of her hot flashes, her irritability, or her forgetfulness. Today, thanks to the work she did to optimize her hormonal communication, she's continued for years symptom free.

# Chapter 10

# STRUCTURAL INTEGRITY

> **Structural Integrity** (from subcellular membranes to musculoskeletal structure)
>
> Structure is intimately related to function and thus to potential dysfunction. The structural integrity system encompasses body structure from the smallest to the largest level. This includes the integrity of organelle membranes, the cytoskeleton, and the cell membrane; the alignment of bones, ligaments, muscles, and tendons; and the structure of all the major organs.
>
> When structural integrity is optimized, body functions such as movement, balance, strength, and cognition can reach their maximum potential, while dysfunctional structures can lead to deficits in these body functions and, in some cases, to severe pain.
>
> Common problems that involve dysfunction in structural integrity include osteoarthritis, osteoporosis, neuropathy, and chronic pain.[2]

Remember Dizzy Dean from chapter 1? He was the baseball pitcher who threw one of his famous fastballs only to have it slammed right back at his foot. His big toe was fractured, and he went back to playing before it was fully healed. As a result, he had to change the way he threw the ball. That altered motion ultimately led to an arm injury that ended his career.

This is a great example of the interconnectedness fundamental to the discipline of functional medicine, but it also illustrates a dysfunction in the seventh area of the matrix: structural integrity. Dizzy Dean's toe injury threw off his body's chiropractic structure, and the subsequent change in motion made a problem pop up in a seemingly disparate area of the body—in this case, his shoulder.

Compromises in structural integrity often work that way—they start a chain reaction that may manifest itself in a way you wouldn't expect. And structural integrity includes far more than the musculoskeletal problems we saw in the story of Dizzy Dean: even at the cellular level, a structure that's somehow broken down or gone haywire can cause major problems. Let's take a quick look at the three levels of structural integrity, starting small and then zooming out.

At the **cellular membrane level**, structural difficulties overlap with the communication system we talked about in the previous chapter. You'll recall that the cell membrane is a layer of fat, and if the fats in your diet tend to be solid at room temperature (as is the case with animal fats), you're going to have stiffer cell membranes. That means that the receptors floating around on the cell membrane are also restricted, causing you to lose some receptor sensitivity. So signaling chemicals—hormones—can be present in abundance, but if the receptors are stuck on a stiff membrane, they won't be able to receive the message. To use our metaphor from the last chapter, you may have plenty of keys, but they're no good if the lock isn't working. The problems that result from this imbalance run the gamut from menopausal problems to diabetes to thyroid malfunction.

Structural integrity at the **organ system level** overlaps with a different area of the matrix, the first one we discussed: assimilation. This is because most structural problems at the organ level start with the gut, the main site of assimilation. When the structure of the gut becomes leaky—when, thanks to chronic inflammation or some other infectious agent, your immune system starts having abnormal interactions with the material that should be contained to the gut—an autoimmune process begins that affects the structural integrity of other organs. Gut leakiness and its resultant antibodies may cause us to develop autoimmune thyroiditis, or the liver may become flooded and its structure weakened. And with all this systemic inflammation, the blood-brain barrier may be affected as well, potentially contributing to a whole host of other problems, including attention deficit disorder and Alzheimer's.

The next level of structural integrity is the **musculoskeletal level**, and this is what we started out talking about with the case of Dizzy Dean. Musculoskeletal health is the primary domain of chiropractic care, which is all about optimizing structural integrity at the spinal level. By ensuring that there is fluid motion in all the joints, the chiropractor prevents the body from focusing stress in any one area of the body, which can cause problems throughout the entire musculoskeletal system. The human body is like an eggshell—the shell is very delicate, but because of its shape, you can hold it your hand and squeeze evenly on all sides without breaking it. Hit it on the side of a pan, though, and it will break right away. When motion in one joint of the body is no longer fluid, you end up with point stress, which is like bringing the egg down on the side of the pan. Imagine, for example, not being able to move your right shoulder properly. You then have to bend at the waist to point the shoulder higher, and by doing that you put more stress on your lower back and end up with problems there. Or if the arches in your feet become stiff or frozen, the energy from walking is transmitted rather than absorbed, and you end up with pain in the ankles, knees, or even hips.

Fortunately, there are ways to optimize structural integrity at each level—cellular, organ, and musculoskeletal. They include changing the types of fat in your diet to promote healthy cellular structure; healing the gut structure with probiotics, nutrients, and dietary changes; and focusing on correcting the first fallen domino that set off cascading problems throughout your joints and spinal system.

◦–◦–◦

From the start of his first visit, it was abundantly clear that Vern didn't want to be in my office. His wife, Joan, had dragged him in by the earlobe.

"Hello," I said as I entered the exam room to find the fifty-something couple sitting side by side in a couple of chairs. "I'm Tom. How are you doing today?"

Joan introduced herself pleasantly, but Vern's greeting was gruff. After grunting hello and shaking my hand, he sat back down and crossed two meaty arms over his paunch. He was moderately overweight, though not quite obese.

"So, Vern, what brings you here today?" I asked.

"She does," he replied, jerking a thumb toward his wife. Joan laughed but rolled her eyes.

"Okay, Joan," I said, smiling to show I saw her annoyance. "Why did you bring Vern in today?"

"The short answer is diabetes," she replied. "He was diagnosed five or so years ago, and they put him on three medications. But he doesn't take them as much as he should, and his diet is terrible. I want to see if you have some way to help him. Not more medications, but maybe something natural."

Vern sat silent and unreadable. "Well, Vern, what do you think about that?"

"I'll do whatever you think will fix me up, but I'm not big on health foods," he said. "She's probably right that my diet could be better, but I'm just a meat-and-potatoes guy. What can I say? It's what I like to eat."

"We can talk about your diet a little later, but why don't you tell me more about the diabetes diagnosis," I said.

"I can tell you that I'm not sure I even believe it," Vern said.

Next to him, Joan gave a long-suffering sigh. "Did you look at the paperwork I brought in?" she asked me. "His blood sugar is high every time they take it."

I had indeed looked at Vern's paperwork from his previous doctor, and Joan was right. His levels were invariably high. In a healthy diabetic, hemo-globin A1c levels should be around 6.5 or 7, and Vern was around 11. "So your blood sugar is very high," I said to Vern, "but you're not sure you believe you have diabetes? Why is that?"

"I just don't . . . I mean, couldn't it just be that I ate a candy bar or something before they took it?"

"Well, not really," I said. "A healthy body would be able to absorb that sort of sugar shock, and it wouldn't register as heightened levels like this. Are you measuring your blood sugar at home?"

Vern gave Joan a sheepish look. "I'm supposed to, but I don't."

"He doesn't take his medicines much, either," Joan added. "That's part of why we're here. I want him to take care of this, but I don't feel right telling him to shovel down pills every day. Our family . . . we don't really trust medication."

"Well, I sympathize," I told her, "but some of those medications could be doing him good, at least in the short term. Our goal will be to get him off them eventually, but you really need to be taking them, Vern. Failing to take them could prove disastrous. I see here that you were referred to diabetic education by your other doctor. Did you go?"

"He didn't," Joan answered. "He wouldn't go."

Vern cupped a hand around his chin and looked to the side, silent. I could tell that getting him to believe what any doctor told him was going to be a challenge—and getting him to comply with my recommendations even more so. "But you are having some symptoms, right, Vern?"

"Well, yeah, but I think it's just prostate problems or a bladder problem. I'm urinating a lot, but I'm pretty sure there are medications that can take care of that."

Vern was displaying a misunderstanding that's common among the diabetics I see. Usually they've seen a million ads touting drugs for frequent urination, and they think a pill will give them a quick fix. But frequent urination isn't just a standalone quirk of bodily functioning; it is often the first noticeable effect of high blood sugar. I had a hunch Vern's diabetes was behind his frequent bathroom visits. "Can you pinpoint for me the last time you felt well?" I asked him. "And I don't mean 'just okay'—I mean truly, wholly well?"

Vern thought for a moment. "I'd say it was several months before I went to the doctor five years ago. That summer I came down with something; I figured it was the summer flu. Body aches, fever, all that—just felt like hell. I eventually got better but never back to a hundred percent. That winter was when it got really bad. I was urinating all the time. I was getting up several times a night. And I was so thirsty. I thought maybe I was eating too much salt, but I was also tired. I just couldn't understand why I felt so drained. But anyway, that's what took me to the doctor for the first time. And that's when they told me I had diabetes."

Vern's story of the suspected summer flu caught my attention, and I immediately suspected it had been the trigger that brought his diabetes symptoms to the fore. In most cases of adult-onset diabetes, the patient slowly becomes insulin resistant as time passes. It happens like this: The patient's diet constantly raises the blood sugar, and the pancreas has to repeatedly produce great amounts of insulin to allow the sugar to enter the tissue. But the pancreas can only make so much insulin. And at the same time, the tissue may become desensitized to the insulin's message, particularly if the cell membranes are stiff—if, in other words, the structural integrity of the cell has been weakened. As a result, blood sugar rises progressively, until it's high enough to be called diabetes. In Vern's case, I suspected this had been happening and that the illness had pushed him over the edge.

Thanks to this flu, his body was overrun by inflammation and his whole system lost a good deal of its efficiency. Part of this would have been a weakening of the pancreas and a resultant drop in the insulin that should be regulating his blood sugar. Combine that with Vern's diet, which was high in the saturated fats that tend to stiffen cell membranes, and you have a perfect storm. Bang—Vern was diabetic.

My guess was that Vern's suboptimal cell structure was preventing the insulin from working as well as it should. Unfortunately, though the insulin struggled to store energy in the muscles, it was still perfectly capable of storing energy in fat cells, especially in certain parts of the body. Like many diabetics, Vern had trouble losing weight and had a good amount of adipose tissue around his waist. The problem was that the insulin's inability to work on muscle meant that even as Vern's body locked up energy in fat cells, it was having to burn muscle for food.

This effect can lead the diabetic to say, "Gosh, I'm really packing on the pounds. I just won't eat today." But the body won't burn much fat during this fast like this person hopes—it will mainly eat up muscle. So perhaps he started at 287 pounds with 30 percent fat and manages to drop to 187 pounds. But then he goes off the diet and regains until he's back at 287. But now he has 33 percent fat, because the insulin in his body isn't working on the right receptors and is storing everything as fat. After another crash diet and regain, he might be at 36 percent fat.

So what's a person to do? The priority—the ultimate underlying problem—lies in structural and communication problems at the cellular level. The structure of the cell membrane is off (it's too stiff), which means that communication between hormone and receptor is diminished. The best way for Vern to start fixing this problem was with what I call an oil change.

●-●-●

Vern and Joan had driven in from a small community in rural Minnesota. He was a farmer, though not in the Old MacDonald mold. He had thousands of acres and a big workforce under him, sort of a CEO in overalls. As I struggled to get him on board with my plan—and convince him that he did, in fact, have diabetes—I tried to use metaphors that would speak to him.

"So think about your tractors," I said. "You change up the oil you put in, right? In the winter, you need thinner oil, because the cold makes it thicker."

"Yeah . . ." said Vern.

"And in the summer, vice versa. You need thicker oil because the heat's going to make it thinner."

"Right."

"Well, your body's kind of like that. The type of oil, or fat, you put in affects the way you run. If you neglect your tractor, you just have to buy a new one. That's not an option when it comes to your body. So we've got to start paying attention to the oil you're putting in. Over most of your lifetime, the fats you've been eating have given you these progressively stiffer membranes. Mother's milk is very high in the right kinds of fats, but then you went to cow's milk and then to fried food and all that, and your membranes started getting less and less able to respond nimbly to the demands placed upon them.

"As your system becomes stiffer in general," I continued, "communication goes poorly and structural integrity starts to fall apart. You become more resistant to your own insulin. That allows your blood sugar to drift up a little bit. Because your blood sugar is up, your insulin comes up to compensate, so now you have slightly high insulin level. Then at some point, you become resistant to your insulin to the point where it starts to drift up and your insulin goes up again. Just before you got that virus, you were probably pretty close to maxed out on your ability to make insulin. Then that illness increased inflammation and decreased your pancreas's ability to make insulin. All of a sudden, your blood sugar can rise unchecked, and now you have diabetes."

Joan was hanging on my every word, as she had been from the start, but by the time I was delivering Vern's story to him, he'd had a few light bulbs go off and was beginning to believe some of what I was saying.

"So Vern, we've got to make some fundamental changes in your diet. Once we get you eating healthier fats—especially omega-3s—you're going to make your receptors a lot more sensitive, and you're going to start fixing some of the fundamental problem here."

"I just . . . I don't know what this means I'm going to be eating. I'm not going to spend the rest of my life munching on lettuce and celery sticks," he added, almost defiantly.

"Well, you certainly won't have to do that," I said, "but it will be a challenge. Changing the way you eat is hard, but you've got to remember the primary reason we eat. What do you think it is?"

"For energy, I'd guess," Vern said, mildly irritated.

"That's certainly one reason. And of course food tastes good, and we get hungry. That's another reason. But we also eat food to get spare parts that our bodies use to repair themselves. Without the nutrients we get from food, we'd totally break down. You fertilize your fields, right?"

"Of course I do," said Vern.

"Why do you do that?" I asked.

"'Cause I'm trying to get a good yield per acre."

"So you're telling me you fertilize your fields so crops will grow better."

"Yeah. That's right."

"Well, think of your diet as a way of fertilizing yourself. Right now, you're planting seeds in the same old worn-out, unfertilized dirt, and it's not doing you any good."

Vern tilted his head back and froze, staring straight at me. After a couple of moments of silence, I was convinced he was about to stand up, say "Hell with you," and storm out. But when he spoke, his tone was calmer than before.

"Okay. I see what you mean."

Beside him, Joan smiled, looking relieved.

"So what kind of fertilizer am I going to have to eat?"

"Well, we could start with cow manure," I said.

Vern laughed but looked a little worried.

"Kidding, kidding," I said. "For that, let's go talk to Danielle."

●-●-●

Danielle, our lifestyle educator, would be the one to go over the nitty-gritty of Vern's dietary changes, but I took her aside before we went over that with him in his first visit.

"Listen, Dani," I said, "this guy is resistant, so we're going to have to start slowly if we want to get him on board. Let's try to give him some things to *add* to his diet rather than telling him all the stuff he *can't* do. We'll save the shall-nots for later."

As we went over how Vern could start giving his body the nutrients and healthy fats that would improve his cellular structural integrity, we tried to keep things simple. The only big "no" we gave him was trans fat, which has been taken out of most food supply now, and excessive saturated fat, which is comprised of animal fats. Other than that, we started with simple add-ons to what he was already doing.

The first thing we added was a vegetable and low-glycemic-index fruit (in other words, one that wouldn't send his blood sugar soaring) with lunch and dinner. Each of those would be two servings, putting him at eight servings of fruits and vegetables a day. Vern typically didn't eat breakfast, and we didn't expect him to start preparing something extravagant each morning. So we just asked that he eat a certain medical food that is specially designed to help with blood-sugar control. We also put him on a fish oil supplement to help with his blood sugar and gave him some supplements. When you have high blood sugar, it acts like a diuretic, and the frequent urination causes water-soluble vitamins to be wasted. So we wanted to make sure he had sufficient magnesium, potassium, B vitamins, and electrolytes.

Dani finished up with some guidelines about portion control, calories, and glycemic load, but she kept it all pretty light and didn't give him a calorie count or anything like that. We just wanted to get him thinking, to gently nudge him in the right direction. We scheduled a follow-up for three months later, hoping to see some improvement then.

"I know you want him off those meds, Joan," I said at the end of the visit, as the two of them pulled on their coats. "But you've got to keep him on them for the moment. We may get there eventually, but if he drops them now, he'll accelerate himself down the track he's on right now—and it's not a good one."

⚫-⚫-⚫

Over the next three months, Vern had a weekly call with Dani, in which she encouraged him to make better and better decisions. By the time he and Joan came in for the first follow-up, he'd succeeded in making some small but significant changes. He hadn't cut out all the big offenders from his diet, but he'd upped his fruits and vegetables and cut back on high-glycemic-index foods, even swapping his beloved potatoes for sweet potatoes (which, oddly enough, have a lower glycemic index than white potatoes). As a result of this, he'd lost about five pounds and lowered his blood sugar by ten points or so—nothing dramatic, but still good progress.

At the second visit, we felt Vern was ready to take on a little more to improve his health. He was still clinging to his blustery ways, though, and I could tell work was stressful.

"There's a big difference between a diet and a change in lifestyle," I told him. "And you're not on a diet. A diet is cosmetic. What we're trying to do is change the whole framework you operate with. We want to make a permanent change. If this were just about a diet, you'd get off it eventually and gain everything back.

"A lot of lifestyle change comes down to attitude," I continued. "Right now, you're holding your medicine in your hand and saying, 'God, I hate this. I do not want to take this medicine.' And then you swallow it. Imagine what would happen if you held the medicine in your hand and said, 'Thank god for the opportunity to take this medicine so I don't have as great of a risk of having all of these bad health outcomes.' After a while, you'd start looking forward to taking that medicine."

Vern kept up his armor but seemed willing to listen.

"You can even change your attitude toward your food," I said. "I know the idea of eating broccoli probably doesn't excite you"—Joan, who had accompanied him again, broke in with a laugh of agreement—"but even that you can learn to actually, sincerely like."

"That may be a ways off," Vern said, "but we'll see."

Over the next three-month period, Vern threw himself into his lifestyle change. To be clear, this had very little to do with me. The concepts I was sharing with him weren't part of some groundbreaking system I came up with. Instead, we were merely helping push Vern to a place where he finally found within himself the motivation he needed to change. He was already primed when he came to my office. His primary care physician had given him excellent healthcare, and his wife and doctor constantly reminded him of the dangers of his condition, all the way up to blindness and heart attacks. The simple tools we provided simply gave him the last little boost to change—and he was ready to change, as we saw in dramatic fashion on Vern's second follow-up.

After three more months, Vern had lost twelve more pounds. And although his blood sugar had been consistently at around 300 before, he was now down to 99—and 100 is normal. The highest point he'd been at over the previous three months was 120. He attributed much of this success to learning the tenets of the paleo diet—something Dani talks to many of our patients about. Adherents of the paleo diet eat what we guess our ancient ancestors ate. The theory is that meat, fish, vegetables, and fruits are the foods we evolved to handle best, and that the abundance of grains in the modern diet can cause harm in some—in Vern's case, high-glycemic-index foods were likely contributing to his diabetes. The paleo diet is an extremely low-glycemic-index eating plan, and Vern had dived into it headfirst. The results spoke for themselves.

But Vern's biggest success was his change in attitude. Before, Vern had felt like he had to elbow his way through every day, and he'd been frequently cranky with his colleagues and with Joan. Now, however, his energy level was through the roof, and his mood showed clear improvement.

"This is the guy I married!" Joan told me. "His supervisors notice it, too. They say he used to come in snorting and shouting, calling people out for not doing their jobs well enough. Now he's smiling and slapping them on the shoulder and telling them they're doing a good job—and motivating them positively when they aren't. It's incredible!"

Vern sat by her as she spoke, looking a little abashed but also clearly proud of his progress, too. The marshmallow under the tough, cantankerous exterior was finally starting to show through.

"I've been exercising, too," Vern told me. "I ride my bike between worksites nearly every day. That's at least a few miles per day. The guys still give me crap when I ride up. They're used to seeing me on my Harley or in the pickup, but . . . it's worth it. I can take a few jokes about bells and baskets."

It was clear that Vern had seen the light, and he wasn't going back. At that visit, I cleared him to get off one of his three medications—the diuretic that had been primarily intended for the edema in his legs. Thanks to the changes he'd made, the edema was now gone.

"Okay Vern," I said at the end of this third visit. "I want you to just keep up what you're doing. Remember that your red blood cells, which are among the shortest-lived cells in the body, live for a hundred and twenty days. So you haven't even had a full turnover since the last time we talked."

I wanted him to keep it up, to give his body the chance to continue repairing itself—including the structure of his cell membranes. I had no doubt that he'd managed to make them less stiff, and that that played a big role in his transformation. As patients like Vern change the oil in their bodies, insulin sensitivity improves, blood pressure lowers, weight lowers, and joint pain reduces. Everything improves because they've dealt with the underlying condition.

At nine months in, Vern came back. He was a little more subdued this time, though he'd lost six more pounds, kept his blood sugar down, and was off the first of his three medications.

"I think I may have been a little . . . high on life, last time," Vern said. "I'm still enjoying it, but it's harder now. It takes more discipline. I've really had to dig in. There's no chance I'm going back, though."

"Great," I said. "And you're exactly right. There's no miracle happening here. It's going to be slow at times—you can work harder and harder and still be going in the wrong direction, but at this point, I think we've got you on the right path. You're working smart. And that work is already paying off."

"The worst is when someone brings donuts to work," said Vern. "I get in such a bad mood having to say no to that."

"Trust me, I get it," I said. "When I was in med school, I got in the habit of having a Snickers and a Coke every day. After doing that for three years, I realized I—a previous marathoner!—was turning into a fat guy. I decided to switch to an apple and tea instead, and it was not easy. Walking past that Snickers bar every day was horrible. At first, I felt like Dr. Strangelove strangling himself. Every now and then, I'd try one again, and it would taste sickeningly sweet after not having it for so long. I wasn't enjoying it, but my brain remembered it as something I liked, so I'd eat the whole thing."

Vern laughed. "Oh man, you're so right. I took a bite of donut a couple weeks ago, and it tasted so sweet it was ridiculous."

"Right!" I said. "If you've trained yourself to think an apple is sweet, a donut is going to be insanely sweet. But I know it's a struggle. Just remember that this is going to become your new normal. You've just got to push through the hard parts. Fake it till you make it. And you will make it."

At subsequent visits, Vern continued to show commitment to his new lifestyle. We had fewer motivational conversations and tended to spend our time trading war stories about how we got through tough temptations.

One of Vern's big insights was that he didn't have to order off the menu when he went out. He was a big character in his small town, and all the waitresses knew him at the diner in town. When he went out with his buddies for a meal, he'd learned to scan the menu and then ask for a mix of healthy foods, even if it wasn't explicitly offered.

"Any place you go is going to have a chicken breast and vegetables," Vern told me. "You just have to ask them for what you want." Now he could go out for a meal with Joan or the guys without feeling totally deprived.

Eventually, we got Vern off all his medications through diet and lifestyle alone. Joan was ecstatic to have him prescription-free. It was certainly no miracle cure—it took nearly a year and half of smart work for Vern to get where he wanted to be. But through the changes he made, he was able to repair himself on a cellular level. With the structure of his cell membranes optimized—and, therefore, communication improved—Vern had put his body back in top working order.

# Chapter 11

# MENTAL, EMOTIONAL, AND SPIRITUAL FACTORS

**Mental, Emotional, Spiritual**

At the center of the physiological systems and the personalized lifestyle processes rests the patients themselves and their integrated sense of well-being—specifically, their functions of cognition and emotional self-regulation as well as their sense of self-efficacy, personal life meaning, and spiritual purpose. The patient's inner life directs the narratives contained in the timeline and the downstream physiological processes addressed in the seven other nodes of the matrix. The choices the patient makes and has made in the past, described in the personalized lifestyle factors, emerge from this central focus.

The therapeutic partnership between healthcare provider and patient evolves from the primacy of the mental, emotional, and spiritual wholeness of the patient and acts as the final pathway of evaluation that integrates the three major functional medicine assessment areas:

1. Retelling the patient's story

2. Personalizing the patient's lifestyle factors

3. Physiology and function—organizing the patient's clinical imbalances using the matrix[2]

Roseto, Pennsylvania, once had the distinction of having one of the lowest heart disease rates in the country. In the mid-twentieth century, it was a rural town, populated primarily by descendants of Italian immigrants. After noticing a near total absence of heart attacks among Roseto's residents, researchers couldn't help but be intrigued by this seeming anomaly, and they decided to see just what made this little town so heart healthy. Could it have been the residents' diet? That was one of the first hypotheses, but after controlling for this and all the other variables they could, the researchers emerged with a very different idea: the answer, they said, was the social connectedness of the group.

At the time, the village of Roseto was made up of a group of families that were bound tightly together by tradition and common beliefs. Multiple generations lived in each home, and the entire town observed the same rituals, even eating the same meals on the same days—spaghetti on Tuesdays, fish on Fridays, and so on. Each villager knew where he or she fit in the stable, reassuring framework of the town. Because of this predictable and supportive societal fabric, stress levels in Roseto were remarkably low—along with heart disease rates.

The functional medicine matrix, as you've seen, is in the form of a circle, with the seven areas we've talked about so far—assimilation, defense/repair, energy, biotransformation/elimination, transport, communication, and structural integrity—forming the perimeter. In the center of this circle sits the beating heart of the matrix: the mental, emotional, and spiritual life of the patient—the same element that brought Roseto, Pennsylvania, its peculiar levels of health.

This psychosocial component is a great example of how the matrix is holographic, with each piece containing a picture of the whole. Of course, this could be said of every node on the matrix (in my emphasis on the importance of each area, I'm reminded of my sister, who declares that each one of her horses is her favorite as she introduces them to you one by one). Yet in some ways, this component of functional medicine really is the most important.

Just like all our other environmental inputs—including the food we eat and the air we breathe—our thoughts, beliefs, and relationships can either be healing and supportive, or they can be toxic. And when you're struggling with getting this central piece of the matrix on track, you can eat all the wonderful foods and take all the wonderful medicines this planet has to offer, but you likely won't get better. You can become stuck in "dis-ease," even if your diet and exercise regimen is impeccable, because you're fueling yourself with toxic thoughts.

I don't want to give the impression that people think themselves sick. That's not necessarily the case. It's more that we are complex, integrated beings, and the psychosocial part of us directly affects our overall wellness. When we have difficulty in this area, it can manifest itself in negative impacts on our bodies. Even the villagers of Roseto eventually lost their heart-health edge as families became more isolated and suburbanized in the 1960s and 1970s.

We often overlook the foundational role this component of health plays. I have people come in all the time who want to focus on whether their vitamin C supplement is precisely the right kind, but the truth is that the "best" vitamin C costs up to ten times as much as the person's current vitamin C—and is just five percent better. Little details like the type of vitamin C are important, but they are just that: little details. We have to first focus on getting the basic things right—eating well, moving our bodies frequently, and thinking healthy thoughts and maintaining healthy relationships (the latter is crucial to the process). The same people who want to get exactly the best kind of vitamin C might be facing chronic stress and anger or may be managing their relationships poorly. When that's the case, there are bigger—and more difficult—fish to fry. Once we take care of those, *then* we can talk about which vitamin C to use.

Imbalances in the mental/emotional/spiritual sector of the matrix can take many forms. One of the most common is a lack of connectedness with the people around us. In the previous example, we saw the direct effect this can have on our health. Despite the adoration of high-achieving outliers in our culture, humans are pack animals. When we are isolated from our social networks, it negatively affects our health. Study after study shows that isolated people live shorter lives and suffer more illness. All we have to do is look to celebrities in Hollywood and in the music industry. Though millions of fans adore big stars, they often feel cut off socially—in a paradox that's a bit like Coleridge's "Water, water everywhere but not a drop to drink." Perhaps this isolation is one cause of the implosions we see so often in celebrities: drugs, alcohol, multiple affairs, and multiple divorces.

Other people suffer due to a pervasive feeling that the world is out to get them; they are perpetually the underdog. I grew up in a family like this. My parents and siblings always talked as if everyone they knew was in competition with them. The refrain "Those assholes!" was not so much spoken as felt. In a way, my family had an inferiority complex. We were not joyous among our peers; we were fearful. It was a struggle against the odds to achieve, or so it felt to me. That struggle will take you places—sometimes dark places. Shedding toxic ideas and believing in the basic good of life has helped heal me as I've moved forward in life.

Another common problem is people who beat themselves up about every little thing. When I see people like this, I demonstrate their attitude by dropping my pen on the floor. "Oh my God," I say, "how could I have done this! I'm a complete idiot! You moron! I can't believe how stupid that was!" They usually smile in recognition at the internal tirades they give themselves for minor infractions. These people show themselves a kind of animosity and criticism—even over insignificant mistakes—that they would never show a friend. And often they count rather trivial situations, such as mild criticism from a friend, as a major knock to their worth as a person. This constant negative noise has a big effect on both their ability to move forward in life and their physical wellness. The greatest thing a person can do after making a mistake or running up against criticism is to get back up and keep on trying—but the problem is that after someone's been knocked down over and over, it becomes progressively harder to get back up. When I encounter people like this, I suggest they speak to themselves as they would to a close friend, using their most compassionate voice. If you try this, you'll find that you would never say the things you say to yourself to a friend. The goal is to learn to be a compassionate friend—to yourself.

Others are the kind of type-A individuals who are driven not by excitement and curiosity but by fear of failure and a drive for perfectionism. Yet others suffer from self-esteem so low that God himself could descend from the clouds and say, "Thank you so much; what a wonderful thing that you've done!" and their first thought would be *Oh well, I fooled another one; he didn't see all the flaws.* These people will often give and give and give, mostly due to a dislike for conflict and a crippling guilt about saying no. They then feel taken advantage of—all these people are taking from them! But because they created that situation, they lose a sense for what is fair. I ask patients like this to place themselves in the other person's position. In that person's shoes, would you be asking for help? The answer to that question tells you what to do. If you wouldn't be asking for help, then you shouldn't help. Instead, you should point out a way for that person to come to his or her own solution. If you're constantly giving away what's yours rather than showing the person how they can achieve it themselves, you're giving a man a fish and feeding him for a day rather than teaching him how to fish and giving him his own supply of sustenance for a lifetime.

●-●-●

Kara, smart as a whip and fiery as a comet, first came to my office nearly ten years ago. A small-framed woman with closely trimmed blonde hair, she was quite upset on that first visit. She huffed out a whole laundry list of problems that she said were making her life miserable: body aches and muscle pains, chronic dyspepsia, suspected depression, and anxiety.

On that day not quite a decade ago, we went through the full assessment; I did her timeline, showed her the matrix, and retold her story. Her main complaints were GI problems—abdominal pain, gas, bloating, and alternating constipation and diarrhea—and some structural challenges in the form of muscle and joint pain. The workup we did indicated dysbiosis and adrenal insufficiency. But the thing that struck me about Kara was her attitude. When she described her symptoms, it was with a scowl and curtness in her voice that suggested barely contained anger. I had a hunch right away that this outlook itself was a significant part of her problem, but the more immediate issue, it seemed to me, was assimilation. We started with my standard treatment for that, including the elimination diet (discussed in chapter 3) and the five Rs of healing the gut (see chapter 4).

Yet after a few visits, Kara's treatment had shown only a moderate amount of improvement—in truth, less than I'd anticipated. We'd addressed the dysbiosis, and I was a bit mystified as to why her symptoms weren't gone or significantly better. But in that time, Kara started to slowly open up to me, and more causes of her deep-seated unhappiness revealed themselves. She and her husband had adopted their nephew, Mason, a small child who suffered from fetal alcohol syndrome, and were struggling to handle him on top of raising an older son, Rob. Given the somewhat disappointing results of treatment thus far, I listened carefully, figuring that the next step was to address the psychosocial issues underlying Kara's condition. She'd been told by other doctors that her problem was in her head; my job, as I saw it, was to convince her that her head—in other words, the mental and emotional aspect of her well-being—was just another part of the matrix and just as important, if not more so, than the health of any other organ in the body.

"My husband was the one who pushed for the adoption," Kara told me when she finally revealed her situation. "My initial reaction was that this was *way* too much to take on. But he insisted that we make it happen."

"And you feel like he's not doing his part to help raise Mason?" I asked.

"Well, raising Mason isn't like raising any old kid. When he came to us, he'd already had a few brushes with law enforcement. He just can't seem to control his impulses. For the first bit, I felt like Carson and I were handling it as a team, but that just didn't last."

"What do you think changed?" I asked.

"I don't know. But I can't believe the way he acts sometimes. It's just absurd. I'm trying to turn this kid into a functioning, productive member of society, but Carson undermines me almost every day. He acts like I'm some kind of wacko disciplinarian when all I'm trying to do is do what's right for Mason. And like I said—taking on the huge responsibility of Mason, with his behavior and his past, was all Carson's idea." Kara's brow was knotted as she spoke, and she gesticulated wildly to emphasize her points.

"Everyone who knows him seems to think he's perfect. Don't get me wrong, Carson is a good man and I love him . . . but the people in our community don't have to live with him. They don't see how cold and unsupportive he can be as a parent and as a partner."

Based on conversations like these, I could see that Kara's problems likely extended beyond the physiological. Her diet was decent and had improved since she came to me. She was an active person. All her labs came back clean. ("You know, you're in great shape for the shape you're in," I told her once.) She'd even been to the University of Minnesota Medical Center to try and get well. And yet, at appointment after appointment, Kara curtly complained of the same aches and pains, the same gastrointestinal discomfort, the same depression and anxiety.

Based on her general lack of problems in other areas, her failure to respond to treatment, and the negativity I saw in the way she approached her life, I became more and more interested in exploring the center of the matrix. As all functional medicine practitioners know, when a person has a full workup from a place like the UM Medical Center, the Mayo Clinic, or the Cleveland Clinic with no major problems found, it's time to start looking at an area that institutions like this often ignore: the total interrelatedness of the human being, including the person's psychosocial and spiritual states.

Addressing this component of health is a deep art of medicine that has been largely lost, and it can only be relearned when physicians decide to stop taking the easy road when a patient doesn't respond to treatment. It's often tempting in that scenario to blame the patient and say, "He didn't follow my instructions closely enough" or "Well, she probably has Münchausen syndrome—she's just feigning illness for attention" or "Well, he's probably just depressed." Instead, we need to view patients as whole beings, believe them when they say they're ill, and come up with a new test to find the problem, even if it's one that's in the mind, the heart, or the spirit. Doing that requires listening, suspension of judgment, and a healthy dose of compassion.

●-●-●

At each of Kara's appointments, I brought up the psychosocial component at the center of the matrix, each time emphasizing its importance a little more. As I do with all my patients, I was "pinging" her continuously—sending out little sonar blips to see what she was ready to handle.

Patients can vary widely when it comes to readiness to address this component of the matrix. Some are open to it, even eager for it, right away. I had a woman in my office recently who, after I asked a few questions about her parents, revealed, "I'm convinced that most of my problems stem from the fact that I never felt affirmed by my parents when I was growing up." Wow. That was quite an insight.

If I ping a patient and sense that she falls into the category of people who are ready to accept the toll that mental and emotional problems can have on physiological well-being, I'll bring it up within the first few minutes. The sooner any patient sees that an emotional or relational problem may be at the heart of his or her unwellness, the better. That's when real healing can begin.

Other patients are less receptive to this aspect of the matrix, and I can usually sense it early on. With them, I have to move more slowly. I ask, as usual, the same questions most physicians would ask but also carefully start throwing in deeper questions to see how they react. Rather than just asking about the health status and any significant diseases of the patient's mother, I'll ask the patient how her relationship is with her mother. If the patient looks bewildered and reluctant to answer, or challenges me on this question's relevance, I know it's time to move a little slower.

Some patients have a locked and barricaded door between themselves and the root problem that lies in the psychosocial region of the matrix. If I realize that one such patient has a significant problem with abandonment that's exacerbating her state of dis-ease, it won't do any good for me to try to hack down that door with an axe. Instead, I have to go slowly and demonstrate the power of our mental and emotional states. It's not important that *I* know abandonment is this patient's issue; the real breakthrough comes only when she realizes it for herself.

Kara was not the type of patient to jump on the mental/emotional/spiritual bandwagon. But just as I started to gain more of her confidence and convince her that her attitude toward life played a big role in her health—about a year after she first came to see me—a tragedy struck that would throw her even further off course.

⊛-⊛-⊛

About a year after I first met Kara, her hometown was ripped apart in the wake of a horrific high school shooting. Kara's husband, Carson, was a counselor at the school, and though he survived, the experience scarred him deeply.

At her first appointment after the shooting, Kara wept as she recounted the events of that day. Carson had been in the same building—she'd been so close to losing him. But in the months that followed, Kara discovered that maybe she had lost him after all—or at least part of him.

"If I felt like I was losing his support before," Kara told me about a year after the tragedy, "well . . . now I know it's gone." Her look was weary and, as usual, tinged with ire.

"He's been diagnosed with PTSD," she continued, "and I believe it. When we go out to eat, he has to get a table in the corner, away from everyone. I can see him scanning the room for exits, memorizing them. I feel terrible for what happened to him, but . . ." She paused. Outrage and sympathy seemed to be waging war in her head.

"But he's kind of left you out in the cold, huh?" I offered.

"Yes. He has. I feel like he's just checked out of this family. And with Mason, with taking care of him alone . . ."

I could tell Kara was on the verge of tears again. "That must be incredibly hard," I said.

"It is. I feel like I'm looking around me for help, and there's just no one there. But I can't *not* help Mason. It's just not an option to abandon him. It's the right thing to do, and I'm the only person there to do it. For god's sake, Carson is even talking about moving to a different town with our older son Ben just for Ben's hockey season. I'd be alone and the only person responsible for Mason."

It pained me to see Kara in the state she was in, still suffering the aftershocks of such a tremendously life-changing tragedy, but when it came to her own health, it didn't surprise me that her symptoms had come back with a vengeance just as her anger, stress, and resentment levels were hitting an all-time high.

A lot happens subconsciously—beyond conscious decision making—that can either add to or detract from our health. When you have an imbalance in the psychosocial area of the matrix, whether it stems from anger, isolation, lack of purpose, abandonment issues, low self-esteem, or any other number of issues, the resultant negative thoughts are eventually going to take a toll on your body—sometimes in a major way. It was clear to me that Kara's deteriorating attitude and worldview were dragging her recovery down and manifesting as worsening body pain, GI distress, and depression.

In addition to direct physiological effects, our thoughts can also affect our receptivity to the treatment plans that can do us so much good. As I mentioned earlier in the book, I have many patients who come in and want to drop all their pills and "go natural." "I'm on all these medications, and I hate them," they'll say.

"Well, wait a minute—why do you hate them?" I ask.

"I just don't like being on medications," is the usual reply.

"But your goal is to feel good and be healthy again, right?" I ask.

The answer is always yes, and I take the opportunity to describe for the patient two very different reactions to medication. A person could have the attitude described of: *I hate this. I want to get off these pills.* But if you wake up thinking that every morning, how does that affect the rest of your day? How does it contribute to whether you do or don't take the medication?

Alternatively, a person could be grateful for the treatment he is given, whether he go to a functional medicine doctor or a traditional physician. He could have an attitude more like: *Thank God for these medications—they allow me to breathe again* or *What would I do without this treatment? Finally I can spend time with my grandkids again.*

Which of these two attitudes will help the patient be compliant with whatever regimen is prescribed? When patients come to my office, even if their goal is to get off their medication, I am still going to give them plenty of supplements in the form of pills and probably keep them on their medication, at least initially. If they come in mentally and emotionally against them, the treatment isn't going to work.

Some people carry shame about taking pills, and that affects compliance and the effectiveness of treatment, too. *If I'm sick, it must mean I'm too weak to overcome my illness,* they'll think, or even *God must not love me because I have this illness.* These attitudes affect every other part of the patient's life. If you're walking around believing that God doesn't love you, why would you think anyone else could love you? And if you are walking around thinking you're just too weak of a human being to deal with your own illness in a natural way, then how do you overcome any other obstacle in your life?

It's not as if there's a direct, hardwired line between toxic thoughts and, say, GI issues. (Again, it's inaccurate to think a person can think himself sick for years and then think himself better.) But when your worldview is negative, it's going to be nearly impossible for you to beat a path back to wellness.

Sometimes, even a small tweak to the way you view your life can fundamentally change your worldview and therefore your health. One of my patients was a housekeeper at a Christian retreat, and she revealed to me that she had very negative feelings about her profession. Over a series of appointments, we talked through those feelings. We had a long discussion, and I asked her a series of questions about the purpose of the retreat where she worked. At one point, I asked what kind of personal transformations she had witnessed there, and she told a story about a particular marriage retreat. One couple whose room she was responsible for had arrived there broken, but by the time they left, they were renewed and recommitted to their family, and they had thanked her for making their stay so nice. As she told this story, understanding struck like a bolt of lightning—and it changed her forever. She realized that she had created and facilitated a sacred space in which that couple could heal. From that moment on, she was no longer a servant or a flunky. She had been freed from the shackles of housekeeping and was now a person who performed a crucial task: preparing sacred space.

This just goes to show that so much of our psychosocial wellness is about perspective. Are you a garbage collector, or are you an instrument in one of the most important advancements in modern civilization—sanitation? How you view your own situation is entirely up to you. I mean, let's face it: on some level, all of us have trivial jobs. Me? I'm just a family doctor in a small town. I don't work at a world-class clinic like Mayo, and I'm not on faculty of a university. It's my choice whether I dwell on those things or whether I wake up each day to create a sacred space in which people can heal.

⊕-⊕-⊕

At one of Kara's appointments several years ago, she was still struggling—with her physical symptoms, with her anger and frustration, and with the trials of raising her adopted son.

"Mason's in middle school now," she told me. "He still has problems with impulse control and is more than a handful. But he is making progress. He's playing guitar and clarinet now, and he's got a 3.7 GPA. He's a smart kid."

She was clearly proud of him, but her tone was guarded and careful, as if being joyful about his success would bring down more pain on her. As was typical with Kara, even as she spoke about positive things, she folded her arms tightly across her chest.

"You must be excited that he's doing so well," I said.

"Well, yeah," she said, "but sometimes I just can't believe people's reactions. The lady from the county came over the other day to see how Mason was doing, and when she saw how much he'd improved, she acted flabbergasted, telling me it was a miracle and that I should be teaching classes on how I did it. When she asked me how I did it, all I said was, 'I guess by being a bitch.'" She laughed mirthlessly.

"Well, come on, Kara," I said. "You know what they say—men are assertive, women are bitches. But that's not true. You were assertive, and you deserve credit for that." This whole I'm-a-bitch thing was yet another aspect of Kara's self-image and attitude toward the world around her.

"Maybe. But what really got to me was the way this lady from the county was acting. As if I should start sharing how I did it with everybody. Isn't that *her* job in the first place? I told her that she had no idea what was going on in my family and that if I started training other people, I'd only be giving her a free pass to be even more incompetent. It's just absurd, the tiny budget these workers have. They haven't given us even close to what we needed to take care of Mason. They left me out in the cold and now that I've managed to help Mason, they want me to help them, too. It's ridiculous."

Kara was taking all of this very personally. It was as if this county worker had been out specifically to obstruct her. After all these years, she was still full of rage every day—at circumstances, at the growing disengagement of her husband, at her burden with Mason, and at the professionals who hadn't been able to help her.

"Well, look Kara, I think you're coming at this in a way that's not doing any good for you physically," I said, broaching the subject of her worldview's impact on her body once again. Kara had heard this before. At my urging, she already had the Serenity Prayer—our practice's guiding philosophy—attached to her fridge. She had also read *The Four Agreements* by Don Miguel Ruiz (a book I prescribe almost daily to help people with mental/emotional/spiritual problems). "As far as I'm concerned," I continued, "what you're doing is something Mother Teresa—"

"Mother Teresa's one of my heroes," Kara interjected.

"Is she?" I said. "Well, as I see it, there's just one little difference between you and Mother Teresa."

"And what's that . . .?" Kara asked warily.

"Mother Teresa went to Calcutta to the poorest of the poor, and she did it by choice and with gratitude. You're doing similarly selfless work, but you're doing it with spite and with anger."

Kara, looking a little taken aback, crossed her arms tighter and turned her head, thinking.

"At the same time," I continued, "I'd argue that what you're doing is *more* altruistic than Mother Teresa. I'm not detracting one bit from her when I say that, but even though she was helping others, Mother Teresa was still doing what she wanted to do. You, on the other hand . . . you didn't have much choice in this situation. You've been left with this burden you didn't opt to take on. But you're carrying it anyway and doing an incredible job. It's just this toxic attitude you have about it—it doesn't take away from the accomplishments, but it's really taking a toll on your health."

"So you're saying I just need to change my attitude," Kara said gruffly.

"No," I said. "I'm saying that your attitude is the one you chose. Mother Teresa chose an attitude of giving and being hopeful and loving, and—for whatever reason—the attitude you have right now is one of resentment and anger. That is really the only difference between the two of you."

Kara was silent.

"What we have to do," I went on, "is help you transform this anger into an acceptance that this is your life's work. You've done miraculous things with this young man who came into your life, but instead of celebrating them, you're angry and stressed."

I then told Kara, as I often tell patients, that there are two definitions of stress. The first is "the suppression of the nearly irresistible desire to choke the living snot out of someone who desperately deserves it." While I think that one is funny, the next is more useful, and it definitely applied to Kara: stress is caused by doing one thing when you would rather do another. From this perspective, stress is managed by being present with what you *are* doing, not with something else you wish you were doing.

Kara met my eye with a clear, direct gaze. Slowly, her shoulders relaxed. She sighed, and it was as though she had given herself permission to breathe for the first time. "I never really thought about it like that," she said quietly.

As the appointment continued, there was a clear change in Kara. She was looser and more pleasant. It wasn't as if she'd never smiled or laughed in all the years I'd known her, but her facial expressions that day held a relaxed sincerity I'd never seen in her before.

"To be honest with you," she said before leaving that day, "this is kind of life-changing."

●-●-●

Kara's realization didn't solve all her problems. But it was a breakthrough—one that she worked up to on her own.

Since then, I have seen Kara several times. Her negative internal monologue has decreased dramatically, helping her stop living life as if she were in a pinball machine, helplessly battered by flippers and constantly falling into the drain. Instead, her awareness of the way her mental and emotional states affect her health has pushed her toward living more consciously. She has learned to stop being angry with Mason, especially for things that weren't his fault. She has come to see helping this unfortunate young man find success as her life's work. And she has transformed her feelings of abandonment due to her husband's PTSD into feelings of compassion. She came to understand the trauma he'd experienced, and with that understanding came forgiveness. In fact, his ordeal had opened a window for her to the psychosocial realm. In her husband's transformation, she saw the potent power our thoughts and beliefs can have on our bodies. This realization, coupled with the shift in her attitude, is helping her become a healthier person.

At one visit, she came in and said, "It's no wonder I've been hurting so long—I realized I've been folding my arms so tight that my arm and shoulder muscles end up aching like hell. My neck hurts and I get tight all along my back. I just never realized the cause before." She started to connect her frequent knots-in-the-stomach feeling with her feelings of anger and abandonment, too, and once she made that connection, she was typically able to catch herself and stop the cycle.

When we are conscious and mindful of our mental, emotional, and spiritual state, we are fully human; we, like Kara, learn to exercise control in the moment between stimulus and reaction. Everyone I know can benefit from working on this control. A thoughtful, present human being can exercise the full spectrum of human reactions in response to any stimulus. In one context, the reaction might be anger; in another, laughter. Controlling that reaction requires great wisdom.

As functional medicine practitioners deal with patients who have major imbalances in the psychosocial area of the matrix, we work to facilitate breakthroughs like the one Kara had the day we talked about Mother Teresa. Yes, we look at every other area of the matrix and prescribe treatment—all the things described in previous chapters. But a big piece of the puzzle for us is building an open, therapeutic relationship with the patient, and bringing some of the ritual and meaning back to medicine.

When this is done right, the sense of connectedness it creates, and the awareness about our mental, emotional, and spiritual states it encourages, can make all the difference in a patient's healing.

Chapter 12

# INTERCONNECTION

It was just after 8 a.m. on a Tuesday morning in 1996. Paperwork from the previous day's appointments littered my desk when I arrived at the office an hour earlier, but I'd cleaned up most of it. I leaned back in my chair and sipped at my now-cooled green tea, mentally preparing myself for a morning of patients.

Suddenly, I heard a high, muffled cry through the wall, followed by a thumping, pounding, and indistinct voices. I remained behind my desk. I had a hunch it would be like this. After a couple more minutes, the racket died down, and my nurse, Mary Beth, tapped on the door and leaned in.

"We roomed your first patient," she said, pausing to pant for a moment. A strand of hair had freed itself from her ponytail, and she blew it out of her eyes with a puff of breath. "This one's a handful. I got my exercise this morning."

I entered the exam room to a scene of pandemonium. A sandy-haired child of about four lay on the ground, violently pounding the wall with his small white sneakers and shouting at the top of his lungs. A thickset middle-aged woman crouched over the boy, speaking to him in calm tones, while two other adults, who I presumed to be his parents, stood at either shoulder, looking sheepishly on.

"Hello," I said over the child's cries, and the mother turned and walked toward me.

"I'm so sorry," she said, her face pale and creased with worry. "I'm Lisa. When Aaron gets this way, it's impossible to stop him."

Her husband, looking resigned, came over and shook my hand. "John," he said.

"And that's Carol, his caregiver," Lisa said, indicating the woman who was attempting to subdue the flailing boy. I was glad she'd come along—when seeing young patients, I always insist on seeing both parents as well as anyone else involved in the child's care.

Carol nodded a greeting toward me as she continued to work on Aaron. "Come on, Aaron," she said, pulling the boy up from the armpits and putting him in a standing position. He crumpled back to the floor and commenced his spirited kicking assault on the wall.

This wasn't my first time to the rodeo with an autistic child, and we'd furnished this room for just this kind of case—all the unused electrical outlets were covered, and the only furnishings were three upholstered chairs and a simple exam table. We'd even invested the year before in soundproofing to lessen the disturbance to other patients. The only potential trouble spot in the room was the computer, which sat on a desk in the corner and which I'd use to document the visit.

For the next half hour, Aaron remained out of control. At one point, he rushed headlong for the computer, pushing me aside with a shove. Carol ran after him, as did Lisa, and he screamed bloody murder as soon as the two women had his arms and were pulling him away from the machine. He then kicked his mother in the shin and pulled free, darting to the door and beginning to kick it rapidly and repeatedly. John placed both hands gently on his son's shoulders, asking him to please settle down. Aaron offered no response but more tears and more shouting.

A few minutes later, Aaron kicked Lisa again, and she reached down and bundled the writhing child in her lap, cooing in his ear and kissing his cheek even as he batted at her. It was heartbreaking to watch. But instead of showing anger, Lisa motioned for John to bring her the crackers from her purse, hoping that would soothe her son for just a moment. Aaron ate the crackers in his mother's lap, seemingly oblivious to her existence.

For a few moments here and there, Aaron's energy would seem to ebb out of his body, and he'd suddenly look like any normal, cute four-and-a-half-year-old kid. I'd have a chance to speak with his parents and caregiver, and a few times Aaron would even interact with me. After about twenty tries, I finally got him to give me a high five. But then he was at it again, climbing on the table and trying to jump off, diving for the computer, and kicking people and objects indiscriminately. Through it all, he said no words and displayed no clear signs of communication with us adults in the room.

I tried to assure John and Lisa that I understood why this was happening, and that I saw this kind of behavior frequently. For autistic children, routine is vital. They rely on the structure and certainty of events in their day. If a parent takes a detour on the way to therapy due to construction, or even if she slows the car down because there was an accident ahead, it's enough to cause an autistic child distress. So, not only was Aaron not doing what he'd expected to be doing this morning, but also his parents had woken him up in the predawn hours to make the two-hour trip from the Twin Cities to my office. To Aaron, this place was a vastly upsetting new world.

After nearly an hour of observing Aaron's state and his interactions with his parents and caregivers, it became clear that I'd need to remove the child from the situation if we were going to get any real communication done. In a rare quiet moment, I pulled Carol aside. "Do you think you could take him for a walk outside?" I asked.

"Oh, of course," she said, concerned and motherly. She got him out of the room without too much of a struggle. Aaron showed no concern about leaving his parents behind.

Alone with Lisa and John, the situation was still difficult. "I'm so sorry," Lisa said, wearily, her eyes slightly red.

"Really, it's fine," I assured her. "It's not your fault, or his."

"Thanks, Tom," John said. "We know that's the truth, or at least we know that rationally. But it's still hard, and embarrassing, to be honest. When Aaron leaves the house, it has to be with both of us. If we take our eyes off him for even a second, he's gone. He'll just vanish. And when he has a meltdown like the one you just witnessed . . . well, you should see the looks we get."

Lisa nodded. I could see in her face that she had accepted this struggle with her son as the harsh reality of her life. For her, this was just the way life was. "It's awful. We love him, but it's awful."

"I get it," I said. "Having people judge you for what they think is your inability to control your kid—that stigma on top of dealing with Aaron yourself, I completely get how hard it must be. Trust me, I've talked to lots of parents who would understand just how you feel."

John put an arm around Lisa. "Thanks, Tom," he said. They looked exhausted.

"All right," I said, propelling my roller chair over to the computer desk and tapping a key to bring the screen to life. "Let's start from the beginning. Can you tell me when you first started noticing that Aaron might be different?"

Lisa looked at John. "A year and a half ago or so?"

John nodded. "Yeah, maybe a little more. I'd say it was around two and a half that we started noticing."

"Yep. We knew all the milestones," Lisa said. "Like the things kids are supposed to do at certain ages, because of our older two kids—Ally is ten now, and JD is seven—they were both so easy, everything by the book. Both model students, straight-A kind of kids. Aaron was the same, for the first two years. He was saying words at one, played a lot with Ally and JD, but then after he turned two, he just got more . . ."

"More withdrawn," John filled in. "It was hardly noticeable at first, but then it became very noticeable. He stopped talking almost altogether and lost all interest in his brother and sister."

"I thought maybe we were going crazy, but I just started taping him with our camcorder even more than we were normally," Lisa said. "He just wasn't the same kid anymore. Soon we both agreed he had to see a doctor. In the earliest videos, he's laughing and playing with Ally and JD, but if you watch the later recordings, it just tapers off. If you see these videos, you're seeing him lose his speech month by month. We boiled down two years of his life into a couple of minutes, and it's just awful to see the progression."

"Do you happen to have those tapes with you today?" I asked.

John and Lisa instantly looked at each other. "No," she said. "We got so used to doctors not wanting to see them that we just leave them at home now."

"Huh," I said, tapping on the keyboard. "Did they say why?"

"Guess they just didn't have the time," John said, "or thought they saw everything they needed to see just by looking at him."

"Well, do me a favor and bring them in on your next visit," I said. "I understand the pattern you're describing, but I'd still be interested in seeing it myself."

"Will do," said John.

"Now tell me how that first doctor's appointment went," I said.

"They pretty much told us we were worried over nothing," said Lisa. "They told us he looked normal and that everything was fine. So we went to a different pediatrician for a second opinion and heard the same thing. Went back to that same one after six months with even more problems manifesting in Aaron—still they told us they couldn't find anything. Finally we said 'Heck with you guys' and took him to a pediatric neurologist, but he told us the same thing—that we were being hypervigilant, and we should go home and stop worrying so much."

"But he has been officially diagnosed as autistic, right?" I asked.

"Yes, he has," Lisa said. "About a year ago, after we were seeing absolutely no improvement, we took him to another place that specializes in autism. They didn't want to see our videos either"—here she laughed, a little bitterly—"but they did find that he was autistic."

"Not that that helped anything," John added. "It pretty much just got worse from there. He started getting aggressive, like that demonstration you just saw. He stopped talking altogether. He barely slept."

"He lost bladder function," Lisa added to the list. "That's been one of the worst things. He . . . well, he's, uh, finger painted with the contents of his diaper a time or two . . ."

"Oh, and it's impossible to go anywhere with that kid. We have to watch him like a hawk. He'll bolt the second you take your eye off him. We've been in the middle of the Mall of America and before we knew it, he'd taken off into the crowd. We've found him curled up in people's laps or hanging halfway out a window. No fear of strangers at all and no sense of self-preservation."

"And he's on medication?" I asked, still typing.

"Yes," said Lisa. "One to calm him down during the day, one to help him sleep at night. They've even got him on ADD drugs, though we don't think he has ADD. And I'd say these medications aren't improving a whole lot."

"Just marginally," John agreed.

Lisa sighed. "We just want to do what's best for him. We worry constantly about what's going to happen to him . . . you know, down the road . . . when we're no longer around."

Even back in 1996, I'd seen many parents in similar situations. This family had a long, hard journey ahead, but I knew it was one worth taking.

*   *   *

John and Lisa had already started treating their son's autism by going to the autism center and starting Aaron on medications. But as you've seen through the previous chapters in this book, the traditional approach of making a diagnosis and then treating the patient's symptoms rarely results in deep, complete healing. And with something like autism, the diagnosis—the *what*—is almost meaningless unless you understand the underlying *why*: the root cause of the problems.

In fact, almost any disease is like that. It doesn't matter what you "have." What's important is what's underneath the diagnosis. What are the underlying biochemical issues? What events in your past may have triggered the problems? What environmental factors may be contributing to it? And how do your lifestyle and worldview affect it? These are, of course, the questions that the functional medicine approach helps us answer—and once we know the answers, we can set off on the path back toward wellness.

So far in this book, I've discussed each area of the functional medicine matrix in its own chapter. Along the way, I've pointed out many times that despite this separation into chapters, the entire matrix is deeply interrelated. Problems in one sector can be intimately involved with problems in another, and a person can only make progress toward wellness by taking a holistic view of the matrix. That's why I wanted to finish this book with Aaron's story—it's a great reminder that unwellness may manifest itself primarily in one or two sectors of the matrix, but we have to look at the entire matrix for the complete picture.

Let's examine how Aaron's diagnosis of autism looked when I mapped it onto the matrix. Indeed, it had the potential to show up in nearly every sector:

- **Assimilation:** Assimilation is about assimilating our environment into our bodies, which is largely done in the gut. Almost every autistic kid has significant GI problems, including gut inflammation, and Aaron was no exception. He had chronic diarrhea that alternated with constipation and abdominal cramping and discomfort.

- **Defense and Repair:** The inflammation of Aaron's gut also qualified as a problem in this sector of the matrix, which deals with the body's attempts to defend against foreign invaders and repair from injury. When this process goes wrong, the result is chronic inflammation, something Aaron was almost certainly suffering from.

- **Energy:** Many autistic kids have trouble with mitochondrial function—in other words, not effectively turning food into energy. I suspected this function was suboptimal in Aaron, though we'd have to see.

- **Biotransformation and Elimination:** This was one of Aaron's major problem areas. I suspected that he had a metallothionein abnormality, as is common among kids diagnosed with autism, which means he wasn't able to detoxify heavy metals and other persistent organic pollutants. We would indeed soon find that Aaron had high copper, lead, and mercury levels, coupled with low zinc levels. I also suspected that his body wasn't effectively breaking down casein and gluten, and this was resulting in the creation of substances that were adding to his difficulties.

- **Transport:** This sector, which deals with the movement of molecules within cells, between cells, and throughout the body, was fairly clear on Aaron's matrix.

- **Communication:** Aaron was a profoundly picky eater. John and Lisa told me that his diet consisted primarily of chicken nuggets, french fries, and candy corn. Problematically, that meant he was getting a lot of trans fats, which tend to stiffen cell membranes and impede communication—the signaling within and between cells. In addition, he was having trouble with another crucial aspect of communication: methylation, which is the process of converting substances so that they can be detoxified and passed out of the body (and this relates back to the biotransformation and elimination sector). Aaron also had many nutritional inefficiencies, meaning that his body simply wasn't able to effectively utilize many vitamins.

- **Structural Integrity:** The stiff cell membranes that stifled Aaron's communication ability are another example of structural integrity. With the cell structure compromised by this stiffness, the receptors can't float around and effectively communicate with the rest of the body.

- **Mental, Emotional, and Spiritual:** And, finally, we come to the psychosocial realm, which for Aaron was just horrific. Being so young, it was hard to say what the effect was on him around the time of his first visit, but his condition had certainly eradicated his social life and strained his relationship with his whole family. Certainly, the psychosocial state of the family deteriorated, too. John and Lisa frequently felt stressed, and Aaron's brother and sister were inevitably shortchanged of parental attention due to the care Aaron required. When Aaron was dashing through the house, seemingly hell-bent on harming himself, Ally and JD's homework, extracurricular activities, and simple desire for attention and affection had to take a backseat.

As you can see, the diagnosis of autism spans nearly every corner of the matrix, and so it is with many other diagnoses, from fibromyalgia to Alzheimer's, from IBS to arthritis. Though these diseases may show up primarily in a few main matrix sectors, they penetrate deeply into the interconnected systems of body, mind, and spirit.

To a functional medicine practitioner, the traditional diagnosis hardly matters. We look beneath the diagnosis, to the underlying biochemical issues, to the person's past, environment, and overall mindset. So if you come to me with fibromyalgia, I'm not going to recommend antidepressants, anti-inflammatories, and a little bit of yoga. Instead, I'm going to help you figure out *why* you have fibromyalgia and how we can address the cause through diet, lifestyle, and perhaps some medication. By the time we've treated your detox systems, your inflammation, and your dysbiosis, your fibromyalgia is already on its way out the door—all without actually treating the "fibromyalgia."

In this way, functional medicine operates independently of a person's diagnosis. All the diagnosis represents to us is a final result of something else. Based on your genetics and an infinite array of triggers, antecedents, and mediators, a set of problems in the matrix could lead to a vast array of diagnoses: heart disease, diabetes, thyroid disease, menopause, you name it.

And yet, no matter what label we give the disease, no matter how the dysfunction manifests, it always comes back to optimizing the matrix functions.

●-●-●

"In a lot of ways, autism—and a lot of other conditions—are like the diseases of days gone by," I said to John and Lisa on the day of their first visit. They sat across from me, giving me a deer-in-the-headlights stare. They were clearly still somewhat traumatized by the morning's ordeal with their son. Nevertheless, I wanted them to understand how we were going to go about helping him and how this approach would be different.

"Back in the early 1900s," I continued, "we had this 'fever' that a lot of people got. Some of them felt sick for a while but ultimately did okay; some experienced little more than brief discomfort; others died from it. Must've been pretty confusing back then, but now we know the reality. Some of those people with fever actually had spinal meningitis—they're the ones who died. Some had the flu, and others just had a passing cold.

"That's a lot like what autism is for us today. And Alzheimer's and many other diagnoses. Autism is just a collection of symptoms that we lump together and label a certain way. We're still looking for the equivalent of spinal meningitis and the flu when it comes to causes of autism. Right now, we have a few good hunches, and that's about it. And we certainly don't know all the causes."

"So what does that mean for treatment?" John asked.

"Well, it means that we're going to have to dig deeper than just giving him some pills to help his symptoms. I'm not going to lie. It'll be more of an ultra-marathon than a sprint. But there are a ton of things we can do, and we need to just start on them, one by one to see what works. Some will help Aaron, others won't, even though they might help another kid in the autism spectrum. But we have to do them one at a time, because if we did all nine hundred and eighty-seven at once, it might work—but we'd never know what the underlying problem is."

"Well, if we try something and it's working, do we have to know the problem?"

"If you have the time and resources to implement all those treatments at once, sure—but I'm guessing you don't. Even the one-at-a-time approach is not for the faint of heart. We're going to be exploring Aaron's biochemistry—maybe there are places we can intervene, maybe there aren't. We're just going to have to see."

Our starting point was clear in my mind: I wanted to clear Aaron's diet of casein and gluten. When we digest casein (found in milk) and gluten (found in certain grains, like wheat), our bodies create two morphine-like substances: gluteomorphins and casomorphins. Some people have a problem in the biotransformation and elimination sector of the matrix and lack the enzymes to break these substances down into amino acids. That means that the gluteomorphins and casomorphins can pass into the brain and significantly affect functioning—in effect, it's as if the kid is doped on heroin.

But when I told John and Lisa that I wanted their son to try a gluten-free, casein-free diet, they looked at me like I'd lost my mind.

"Did you hear me earlier?" John said. "All Aaron eats—and this is when we can get him to eat—is chicken nuggets, french fries, and candy corn. Literally, that's it."

"Well, you're in luck," I said. "You can pretty easily find those three items in versions that contain no gluten or casein."

"So we just switch to those versions and keep his diet the same?"

"At first. But of course, that's not an ideal way for him to eat. If he accepts the gluten-free, casein-free versions of his staple foods, I want you to slowly start him on a medical food I'm going to give you. It's packed full of phytonutrients that are going to help him detoxify better and convert his food to energy better."

I swiveled in my chair as the door creaked open behind me. Carol stepped in, steering Aaron before her. He seemed calmer than before, though he still looked mainly at the ground.

"Hi, Aaron," Lisa said, putting on a cheerful tone.

He ignored her, walked over to the exam table, and lightly kicked it. Then he veered left and approached me. He pulled himself up onto my lap, curled up, and just lay there quietly. I knew he was just looking for a soft, warm place to rest—it was no sign of affection—but for the moment, he looked like a perfect angel.

Lisa, John, Carol, and Aaron left that day with full instructions from our nutritionist on the plan for Aaron's diet, and with orders for a NutrEval test—to gauge Aaron's nutritional efficiency—and for a urine test that would test for the heavy metals I suspected he was struggling to detoxify. Those labs would take six weeks, at which point the four of them would return for a check-in.

⚬-⚬-⚬

After a mere month and a half, I wouldn't expect much improvement in an autistic child, but when I next saw Aaron, Lisa and John were thrilled with his progress. After just two weeks of no gluten and no casein, and with only limited nutritional supplementation, Aaron had started speaking, albeit on a limited basis. But he had started repeating things his family members would say to him—his mom might say, "How are you, Aaron?" and he'd parrot back, "How are you, Aaron?" This is known as echolalia, and to Aaron's parents, it was a sign they were moving in the right direction.

In my office for the second visit, Aaron's wildness had abated. When his parents called to him, he responded, and he could even follow simple commands—"Come over here," "Stop doing that," and so on. He still threw a couple of tantrums over the course of the appointment, but they were less intense and shorter than before.

Aaron's urine test showed significant elevation of mercury, a fact that concerned his parents, of course. Today, many are concerned about mercury from immunizations, though that problem has largely been addressed. (And though I'm not anti-immunization by any means—my family and I are immunized—I think the jury is still out on some of the effects vaccines have had on children.) There were plenty of other ways Aaron could be getting mercury in his system, and the problem wasn't the exposure, most likely, but rather the boy's inability to detoxify it properly. If his body failed to detoxify the same number of mercury molecules it was exposed to each day, he could be ending up with a daily net positive of mercury. As that mercury adds up, it can have a serious physiological effect.

Aaron's NutrEval showed even more problems—his body was utilizing virtually no nutrients effectively. He had antioxidants, B vitamins, and minerals that were all inefficient. He also had multiple sky-high markers for both bacterial and yeast dysbiosis—meaning that the good bacteria in his gut was far outweighed by the bad. His ratio of omega-6 fats to omega-3 fats was way out of whack, which meant that the structural integrity of his cells was likely compromised and that his communication system was probably not working effectively. His copper was very high and his zinc very low—which is consistent with metallothionein abnormality.

He also showed signs of methylation defects, though we were already addressing these with the medical food prescribed after the first visit. If we improved the methylation, Aaron's body would do a better job of ridding itself of the heavy metals that we now knew were present in high levels.

Based on this, we recommended that Aaron's parents continue the gluten-free, casein-free diet and the medical food but also add on several other components to the treatment:

- For the metallothionein defect inhibiting his detoxification ability and that had led to the high mercury levels, we put him on **zinc at every meal**. That, obviously, would raise his zinc level but would also block the absorption of copper—one of the other metals he was having trouble flushing out.

- To help further rid him of metals, we put him on a super green food and started him on DMSA (dimercaptosuccinic acid, a metal chelator), both of which would boost his ability to detoxify mercury.

- For his raging dysbiosis, we put him on a **big dose of probiotics** and on **immunoglobulins** that would manage the "bad" bacteria in his gut.

- For his undesirable ratio between omega-3 and omega-6 fatty acids, we gave him fish oil (rich in the omega-3s we wanted to encourage).

Getting a four-year-old to eat all that stuff—especially the DMSA, which, honestly, tastes kind of like rotten eggs—was going to be a challenge. John, Lisa, and Carol and I talked about it extensively, and I suggested they try putting the DMSA in a pocket of peanut butter to see if they could get Aaron to eat it before he noticed the bad taste. I also referred them to a local listserv called BEATMN (Biological Education Assessment Treatment Minnesota), where they could meet other parents of autistic children, some patients of mine, who were working on solutions to the same challenges. When I saw the family off after the second visit, they looked daunted but hopeful. The strides they'd made in the first six weeks were all they needed to keep pressing forward.

At the next visit, six weeks later, Aaron was about the same but he'd started "parallel playing" with his siblings—in other words, playing alone but in their vicinity, which showed he wanted to be involved. His echoing of words said to him was continuing. There was a moment of alarm when I showed John and Lisa the latest urine test—the mercury levels were way up, and now there was cadmium and lead. But I assured them that this was a good thing. It meant that Aaron's body had begun to clear out its backlog of toxins and mobilize the heavy metals, which were now streaming out of his body.

Over the ensuing year, improvement continued. Aaron began saying one-syllable words, then to babble a bit. His meltdowns became less common. He finally got the hang of potty training. He could follow more complex, multi-step commands. All the while, the metals in his urine kept increasing. It is typical for the urine metals to increase, peak, and then fall; the time from the start to the peak is the measure of total burden in the body. In Aaron's case, it was large. He had a lot to get out.

By year two, Aaron's NutrEval and heavy metals tests were looking normal. Now six and a half year's old, he was perhaps not "normal" but more like a high-functioning Asperger's kid than someone with full-blown autism. He was still a little bit of an oddball, but compared to where he came from, that was huge.

◆-◆-◆

Ten years later, I was once again in my office, at a paper-filled desk, when Aaron and Lisa arrived at the office. It was near the end of my day, but when my nurse told me they were here, I instantly smiled—it had been years.

They sat out in the waiting room and both stood when I emerged from the back.

"Tom!" Lisa exclaimed. The lines on her face had spread a bit, but middle age suited her—she looked infinitely better than the weary young mother I'd met so many years ago. Aaron, now a slim teenager with an unruly mane of dark-blond hair, stood beside her.

We chatted for a minute or two, and I learned that Aaron still follows a gluten-free, casein-free diet—though he does allow for a weekly slip-up, and it doesn't seem to bother him. On top of that, he's on a daily probiotic (though not the big ones he was on at first), and he takes zinc and a high-potency multivitamin that does not contain copper.

In a conversational lull, Lisa switched gears: "Well, Tom, we might as well get to why we came to see you. Aaron? Do you want to tell him?"

"Dr. Sult, I'm going to college," Aaron said simply. His smile was restrained—but it was definitely there.

Lisa beamed. "He got bored in high school, so he's actually already taking classes that will count toward college. When he goes off to school next year, he'll enter as a junior!"

I succeeded in holding back tears, but it took some effort. "Wow, Aaron!" I said. "That's fantastic! But . . . are you sure you want to skip freshman year? I heard that one's the most fun."

Aaron blinked and turned to Lisa. "That's a joke, isn't it, Mom?"

"Yes, honey," she laughed.

He turned back to me with a wide grin. "I'm still not so good at that."

●-●-●

Aaron's is an incredible story, and the results aren't always that dramatic. For some kids who come to me like Aaron did on his first day, we use the same process but don't get past the early milestones. And yet, for those parents, it's enough to have their child potty trained and to regain some sense of communication and presence with their son or daughter.

Will science ever uncover the cause of autism and show us a sure, single path to treatment? I doubt it highly, just as we never found a "cause" for fever. Instead, I believe that more and more physicians will recognize that each autistic child is unique and complex and that there may be several different causes of the condition we currently call "autism."

This would be a move toward what functional medicine already does for patients with autism or with any other chronic problem. When any doctor, functional or traditional, steps back and sees the whole picture, to seek the *why* and not just fix the *what*, the therapeutic relationship between healer and patient is restored. It's clear that we'll never have all the answers or be able to cure all the world's ills. But functional medicine is nevertheless at the vanguard of a movement that I believe will transform healthcare as we know it.

Perhaps one day, it will be standard to look straight to the heart of sickness and disease rather than trying to throw a bottle of pills at a few symptoms. Perhaps one day, mainstream physicians will recognize that chronic diseases require a radically different approach than the one they currently take—one that looks for connections rather than isolates problems and seals them off into categories. Perhaps one day, doctors will have time to sit with patients, to get to know them as people, and to understand the crucial links between their health and who they are as people.

Until then, functional medicine will continue forward, touching patients like the ones you've read about in this book. This is not to say we are miracle workers. Some of our patients are too sick to recover. Many don't recover to the degree they'd like. But we can offer patients honest, open-minded, intellectually curious, relationship-based, holistic treatment that—if it works like it should—brings them insight, healing, and most important, hope.

# Chapter 13

# WHERE THE MAGIC HAPPENS

As any one of my patients will tell you, applying the principles of functional medicine to your life isn't exactly a walk in the park. It's simple, yes, but that doesn't mean it's easy. Patients don't walk into my office, listen to me talk for a few minutes, pick up a prescription at a pharmacy, and hope for the best. Instead, they find that I ask them lots of questions—even uncomfortable ones—and that I push them to make changes to the very way they think about living life. If they can make those changes, they become active participants in their journey back to wellness.

Of course, not all patients leave my office after the first visit and comply one hundred percent with my recommendations. Very few can pull it off right away, even if they trust that the treatment I've recommended will heal them. People slip, eat things they shouldn't eat, get too stressed about something they can't control, pick TV over a brisk walk three nights in a row. That's natural; I don't expect my patients to be straight-A students one hundred percent of the time. In fact, I tell patients that if they can just do what I ask them to do *90* percent of the time, in all likelihood, they'll still find themselves on the road to good health.

But sometimes a patient's failure to follow a treatment plan goes beyond the occasional slip-up. Fairly often, a person has significant obstacles to following through, and if that's the case, no number of appointments will move that patient toward wellness. Those obstacles have to be addressed first.

The field of medicine overall has a very high noncompliance rate—the World Health Organization estimates that, in developed countries, only about

50 percent of patients with chronic diseases follow their physician's treatment instructions.[7] When most traditional doctors are faced with a noncompliant patient, their typical attitude is *Oh, well. Too bad that person didn't follow my advice.* Even "holistic" practitioners can put the blame on the patient. One of my biggest pet peeves is seeing a patient who says, "Yeah, I went to so-and-so, he's a holistic doctor, and I did *almost* everything he told me to. He asked me to go on a gluten-free diet, but I messed up and ate gluten once. He said that was the reason his treatment didn't help me." *That* was the reason? Really? Shouldn't the physician have some responsibility in setting the patient up for success?

In my opinion, letting a patient believe he or she is the reason the treatment plan did not work is a cop-out on the part of the physician. It's an easy way of pushing away the blame for a failed treatment, but it does nothing to help the patient. The functional medicine approach is different. My philosophy is that if one of my patients doesn't get better, it's *my* fault. (That's not to say I'm a pushover. In fact, most of my patients will say that I'm kind of tough. Often patients will come in having managed to reach a goal; I'll give them the pat on the back they're looking for and then say, "Wonderful! You won the pennant, but we're after the World Series.")

At the heart of functional medicine, as you've seen in previous chapters, is the therapeutic relationship between physician and patient. What traditional medicine misses is the fact that it's the physician's job, not the patient's, to create context and meaning behind the treatment, and to foster an environment that encourages shared responsibility.

The therapeutic relationship and the retelling of the patient's story are both important to achieving this environment. If I've fully laid out how the patient got from ease to dis-ease and what the path back to ease looks like, the patient will likely leave my office ready to do whatever it takes to get well, even if it's going to be a struggle. So, when a patient goes home and does virtually none of the things I've asked him to, it's for one of two reasons: either I didn't do my job in the first place (I didn't collect the data well enough, I didn't tell the story well enough, or I didn't explain the treatment well enough), or something prevented the patient from doing what he knew he needed to do. Usually that

---

7   World Health Organization, *Adherence to Long-Term Therapies: Evidence for Action*, www.who. int/chp/knowledge/publications/adherence_full_report.pdf.

*something* is deep-seated and important to the patient. If I determine that the latter is the case, my new job is to figure out what that obstacle is.

## WILL THEY OR WON'T THEY?

In the old days, young and testosterone-crazed, I just plowed through my spiel with an attitude of "Hey, I'm busy. You came here to see me, and this is what I think you should do. Now just freaking go do it!" That was really successful—for a tiny percent of my patients. But it was definitely not successful for a very large percentage of patients. As I've grown as a human being, I've realized that when I start meeting even the smallest amount of resistance—"one ping only," as Sean Connery says in his dramatic line from *The Hunt for Red October*—it is much better to stop and explore than to push on through the appointment.

After seeing patients year after year, I've honed my ability to tell very early on who's going to stick with the program and who's going to have issues. If a patient is reluctant or overwhelmed as I lay out a treatment plan, it's crucial that I address this as soon as possible. It's yet another area in which I use the "pinging" technique—I ping the person with a piece of information and closely watch the response, looking for overt or subtle clues to his state of mind.

Some people are pretty obvious about their resistance. They'll say things like, "Hmm, I don't think this is going to work," or "I can't do that." That patient, I know right away, has a very low chance of complying, so it's important that I stop and address his objections immediately. "What do you mean when you say you can't do it?" I'll ask. He'll explain the problem, and we'll start modifying right away.

Other people camouflage their reluctance, and this is where the pinging really comes into play. Maybe I'll notice that "Yes" and "Uh huh" and "Oh, okay!" have turned to "Hmm" and "I see" or even inarticulate grunting noises. Or maybe I see that the patient has gone from leaning forward slightly with eyes wide open to leaning back and squinting at me.

If I get enough of those cues, I'll pause, look the patient in the eye, and ask how she's feeling about everything I've said. Many are good actors, and they'll say, "No, no, it's fine. Don't worry," or "I'm just thinking it through—it's a lot to take in." I follow that by saying, "Well, let me know if you have any questions." But if I continue and am still noticing the telltale signs of resistance, I'll stop and, in my most empathetic tone, say, "Okay, I'm hearing discomfort related to this whole plan. What is going on for you?"

Even then, most people won't admit to the discomfort. They'll say everything sounds good, that they're ready to make the necessary changes. If I'm pretty sure they're feeling intimidated or resistant, I'll stop and say "Well, actually it doesn't seem like it's fine to me, and we are going to be much more successful if we get to the bottom of what you are thinking about."

It's a direct approach, but I try to be as compassionate as possible about it. Every patient wants to get better, but some people just aren't quite ready to open up. I try hard to create a relationship of trust, but sometimes I know that won't happen in the first visit; some people's armor is simply too thick. In cases like that, I know it's going to be a slow process of building rapport and then showing them that the changes I want them to make—though challenging—are the right direction to go if they want to achieve true wellness. They need to see that whatever obstacle they have is worth surmounting and that I'm there to help them through it, whatever it may be.

Over the years, I've heard plenty of reasons why a program won't work for a patient, from the trivial to the profound. Perhaps you've made similar statements to explain why you didn't stick with a regimen you know could benefit you. Let's take a look at some of the most common objections and see how patients can get past them.

## "I TRIED IT AND IT DIDN'T WORK!"

A lot of people will come to the second visit and say, "Well, I did all those supplements, and I did the diet for a couple of weeks, but I just didn't feel that much better, so I didn't keep going."

If you struggle through two weeks of a new regimen and start week three feeling no better than you did originally, it's easy to get frustrated. It's an understandable response, but functional medicine isn't about magic or quick fixes. It's a methodical discipline, and it takes time (despite the wishes of people who've suffered through years or decades of chronic sickness). The body can't rebuild itself overnight.

Remember: a person's red blood cells live about one hundred and twenty days, so simply getting a new crop of red blood cells will take at least that long. It takes patience to see the results of the changes you're making. I always talk about this at the first appointment, but I sometimes have to go through it again at the second or even third visit. Human beings are amazingly good at selective listening. But I keep at it, reminding patients that they have to be in it for the long haul. Change may be slow in coming, but its effects will be lasting.

## "BUT I HAVE NO IDEA HOW TO COOK OKRA!"

It's fascinating how often we get bogged down in specifics and allow one minuscule piece of a program to deter us from the whole thing. For example, I frequently put people on an elimination diet (as described in chapter 3), and I give them materials that lay out all the dos and don'ts and present recipes and menus. One woman had a reaction that's typical of patients who derail themselves by focusing on an irrelevant detail: she'd looked over the plan at home, spotted okra on the vegetable list, and used its presence as an excuse to give up on the whole thing.

When she came back to my office, she said, "I just have no idea how to cook okra. I didn't know what to do."

Pulling out a copy of the vegetable list, I said, "Well, how about broccoli? Or spinach? Okra is one of over two dozen vegetables here." Then, doing my best Tina Turner: "What's okra got to do with it?"

I grabbed my laptop and pulled up Google, as I do at some point in most appointments, and searched "okra recipes." Tens of thousands of results. "And even though you never have to touch another okra in your life if you don't want to," I said, shifting the laptop screen so she could see, "there's a vast number of easy ways to cook okra right at your fingertips. How about this one?"

This woman had created a decoy excuse, which is common for patients to do. Once I point out the flaws in the excuse, the patient may realize that it wasn't the okra that was stopping her, and we address the true obstacle she's facing. But if patients don't have this realization, they're likely to keep on throwing up excuses, perhaps moving to one of the others discussed in this chapter. But there are an infinite number of decoys; I have some patients who, after five years, still haven't progressed too far because of superficial problems with a treatment plan. When that happens, we keep working through it together. If the patient isn't ready to run, I have to walk alongside her.

People who cling to decoy excuses, though, tend to have very little insight into their own psychology. Everything in their world is external to them, but as long as they are unable to understand the internal process of moving toward wellness, they aren't likely to be able to modify behaviors that will allow them to make real change. It is the challenge of the functional medicine practitioner to help them move past the meaningless "can't cook okra" excuses and strike at the heart of their resistance (we'll talk about some of those deeper blocks later in this chapter).

## "KALE MAKES ME GAG."

Another frequent excuse I get is "I don't like such-and-such food." My answer to patients who say this is that they don't have to eat that one food. One guy told me kale made him gag, and when I get comments like this, I point out that millions of other people in the country manage to eat that food without gagging. I wanted him to realize that the gagging reflex is almost certainly psychological and that he probably had a deeper resistance to the program than the taste of a certain food.

Many patients put up resistance when it comes to the taste of supplements, too. This often happens with the powdered drink mixes I prescribe; we use these because it's a way to get a whole bunch of supplements in just one go. Sometimes patients come back and say, "I just can't stand the taste."

"Well," I respond, "it's medicine, not a milkshake! I take it every day. Whether you like it or not, hold your nose and gulp it down."

I also try to emphasize that changing the diet involves reprogramming the brain and the taste buds. In our culture, we tend to think that eating is purely for pleasure, and that can be hard for people to get over. But you *can* change the way you feel about certain foods, especially if you're motivated by health reasons. Taste is malleable and subjective, and people around the world have learned to like some things Americans would find revolting. All you need to do to prove that to yourself is to watch Food Network for a day—or come to Minnesota, where they think lutefisk tastes good!

## "I CAN'T AFFORD IT."

Cost is another common reason patients give me for not following through after the first visit. I've given up trying to tell who's really struggling so much financially that they can't afford the treatment and who's simply using money as another decoy. Some people pull up to my office in a BMW or Mercedes and tell me that the stuff I recommend is too expensive for them, while other people come in by bus and say, "Let's get it done."

One thing I do know: it's usually not about the money. If people are truly balking at the cost of treatment, it's typically because of their perception of the value they're getting. In the car example, maybe the BMW driver thinks, *This is all bullshit and it's not going to work*, while the bus rider thinks, *This is another rock to turn over. Anything that makes me well will be worth it. Let's go.*

Some people don't see the value for what they're paying because, deep down, they're not convinced I'm not a charlatan. There is a voice in the back of their head that says, *This guy is just another doctor* or *He's just some quack*. Or they think I get kickbacks from pharmaceutical companies. I don't blame people for being skeptical. I see it as my job to tell the patient's story well enough that he overcomes that skepticism and is convinced that we're getting him on the path to wellness. If I do that, they'll see the value in paying for treatment.

Plus, all the supplements and other bells and whistles are negotiable. Those add-ons help people get better and feel better faster, but they're not always required. Fundamentally, functional medicine is about diet and lifestyle, and making those types of changes is rarely expensive. It takes effort and persistence, sure, but it doesn't require a fat bank account.

●-●-●

So far, the obstacles we've talked about have been on the superficial side. Most of these are thrown out by the patient in an effort to place the blame on an external cause and prevent the pain of change. These excuses are, as I've said, decoys.

But when I get one of the excuses I've described, it's important for both the patient and me to identify the issue—the real issue—behind the decoy. Because when patients put up roadblock after roadblock to treatment, there's usually a much deeper, more internal element at play: something in their mental or emotional makeup is preventing them from changing. If the problem turns out to be on the advanced side, I might call in a collaborator, like a psychologist. But in most cases, the functional medicine practitioner can use the therapeutic element of the relationship to make some progress on the deeper issue.

Let's look at the two most significant of these internal obstacles—and how you can overcome them should you find yourself up against one.

## EMOTIONAL ATTACHMENT TO FOOD

A few years back, a woman named Amanda came to see me. As we discussed what it was going to take to return her to optimum health, I picked up on some reluctance. Her face fell when I started talking about the foods she needed to avoid.

"I can try," Amanda said after I described what I'd like her new diet to look like. "But it's going to be hard."

"'Do or do not, there is no try,'" I said, pulling out my oft-used Yoda line. So often, people who say, "I'll try" are saying "I'll give it a halfhearted effort and then give up when it becomes inconvenient." But all of us are very capable of doing more than just trying if we put our minds to it.

"It's just . . . certain foods are a comfort to me," Amanda said, averting her eyes from mine. "My mom died when I was eleven, and she used to make me milk toast when I was sick. To this day, I still make milk toast when I'm down. I don't know if I can give that up without feeling like I'm pushing Mom away. Even after all these years."

How could I argue with that? We had identified food sensitivities to milk and wheat, but after her revelation, I couldn't just demand that she cut it out. Losing a parent is a life-altering event at eleven, and here, decades later, she was still soothing the pain with food. I knew we would have to delve deeper.

Amanda's attachment to milk toast is similar to the attachment to food that many of my patients display, even if it's not always as specific or clearly tied to a memory as Amanda's. For some people, food is an antidote to the general stresses, pains, and disappointments of life. They'll say, "Look, food never argues with me. It never lets me down. And it always makes me feel better."

As soon as I sense someone has an emotional connection to food that's going to interfere with compliance, I shift the conversation as far from the food itself as possible. It's just too volatile a subject. Telling someone who's been treating loneliness with donuts "Well, that's it—no more donuts for you!" is about as effective as saying nothing at all. I couldn't just explain to Amanda that all the gluten and sugar in milk toast was contributing to her health problems. Going down that path only creates more resistance.

Instead, I want to start looking at the underlying emotions that drive the patient's actions. With Amanda, it was important to slow down and talk about Mom, about how milk toast had become a replacement for her, about how eating it helped Amanda control her emotions. I had to step back and show that I understood *why* she was eating this way. Once a patient senses that judgment is off the table, we can do more meaningful exploring.

Sometimes I can sense that there's an emotional attachment to food because the person is really stuck on one thing, but I don't know exactly what the attachment is. In that case, I have to do some investigating. If someone says to me, "I did pretty good on the diet we talked about, but every day on my way to work I just *have* to stop at Starbucks for coffee and an apple fritter."

"How come?" I'll ask.

"I don't know," the person might say. "I just have to do it. I can't resist."

This kind of conversation tells me there's something going on and that I need to keep talking about it, but not in a way that's me making the apple fritter the bad guy. "How long have you been eating apple fritters?" I'll ask, digging for the start of the attachment (much as I would when asking the not-well-since question). "How did you feel when you ate your first apple fritter? Tell me about that experience." I try to generate a sense of wonder and excitement about the conversation, striving at all times to stay as far as possible from a tone of judgment.

By taking the conversation down this road, the patient and I are usually able to tie the strong emotions associated with this food to a specific event or phase of life. Maybe the person is trying to remember happier times, like Amanda, or maybe trying to forget a traumatic occurrence in life. As we get closer to that breakthrough, I keep prodding for more information, but as casually, as conversationally, as I can. Assuming the attachment doesn't originate from a tragic event, we're usually chuckling as we talk about it: people realize how silly their devotion to certain foods is, even though that doesn't make it any easier to give them up. Frequently, as we talk about this, the person will stop mid-sentence, look at me, and say something like, "Wow, this still has a lot of control over me, doesn't it?"

Once we get to that epiphany, we're on our way to the discussions that will help us break through where simply forbidding certain foods would have failed. "The important thing is that we keep talking about this," I'll tell the person. "I don't care about the apple fritter. The apple fritter isn't what's killing you, and if you did everything else I asked and still ate the occasional fritter, you'd still make a lot of progress. What I care about are the emotions that seem to be preventing you from moving forward."

Once we start plumbing the depths of the patient's attachment to food, he is much likelier to have breakthroughs—and successfully stick with the treatment plan, where he had failed before.

## LOW SELF-WORTH

Of all the reasons I get for why a patient can't follow my recommendations, low self-worth is the most common. Say a woman comes in, hears what I want her to do, and immediately replies, "Well, there's just no way I can come home from work every night and cook two meals. And I would have to do that. My husband would never eat this way." It's an example of a superficial objection of the "But I don't know how to cook okra" variety—but when I run into it, I know it's likely that the patient's deeper problem is a lack of self-worth.

Why? Well, many people don't make the effort to comply simply because they don't think they're worth it. They don't value themselves and their own well-being enough to possibly inconvenience others as they go about getting better. When someone tells me she can't follow dietary guidelines because of her family, I first tell her about my mom. When my mom was on a diet, the whole family was on a diet, and it worked just fine for us. Nothing I'm recommending will be bad for anyone in her family, so maybe she can prepare a compliant meal and then make just one extra dish for her family that she won't partake in. But after that bit of advice, we often have a bit more exploring to do.

If the patient insists her spouse won't change his eating habits even a bit to accommodate her, I usually ask whether the patient took the time to fully explain the changes she was going to make and how the changes would help her not feel sick all the time. "No," the patient low on self-worth usually says. "It wouldn't do any good."

"So your husband cares more about eating meat and potatoes than about you being well?" I ask.

Unfortunately, that is sometimes the case, though not usually. I'll usually tell the patient that on the next visit, I need her husband to come in, too. Once

I explain to the husband what we're trying to do, how it's going to help his wife, and how she feels about not being able to cook two meals, he'll sometimes say that not only will he change his eating habits to help her out, but—generally to the shock of his wife—he'll also do some of the cooking.

For a patient struggling with feelings of unworthiness, this certainly isn't a final fix. *Sure, he's offered to help*, the patient might think, *but I'll pay for it later*. Even though her husband might be perfectly willing to support her as best he can (or may be dealing with issues of his own that prevent him from helping), she doesn't think she deserves the effort. Bringing the husband in was an important step, but I know I'll need to continue addressing the patient's self-worth issues as we move down the road if she's to have any hope of sticking with treatment in the long term. I'll have to explain that we command the respect we demand, and that many of us demand no respect and therefore command none. This is really about setting boundaries between self and non-self. When a person doesn't draw that line, she begins to think that everyone else's problems are her own and that she has no right to an opinion.

Many women in the situation described have set themselves in the 1950s mold—they see themselves as the family's caretaker, and their own needs go on the back burner. But the phenomenon is by no means limited to women. Men, too, can find that a low estimation of their own value as people can interfere with their ability to stick with the program. Often it's the guy who's a little socially awkward and won't make eye contact who suffers from this. Or, just as frequently, it's the guy who always has a joke ready and takes everything too lightly; his levity is overcompensation for his lack of self-esteem.

Just as a woman might find her traditional societal role impeding her treatment, some men are overwhelmed by the feeling that they're supposed to be successful, strong, and confident. When they feel as though they haven't lived up to this standard of manhood—even if they appear very successful—their self-worth suffers, as does their commitment to improving their health. If a guy doesn't think he's worth anything, if his feeling of inadequacy pervades every molecule of his being, why would he spend three hundred dollars on a doctor's visit and a bunch of willpower on the follow-through?

With patients who suffer from low self-worth, I employ many of the tactics we discussed in the previous chapter. I prescribe books that I hope will change their outlook, primarily *Full Catastrophe Living* by Jon Kabat-Zinn and *The Four Agreements* by Don Miguel Ruiz. We do the "dropping the pen" exercise to reveal just how much they beat themselves up over nothing. And we discuss talking to yourself as you would a close friend—someone they would never criticize as sharply as they do themselves. This last one especially, talking to yourself in a compassionate voice, is often a very revealing exercise.

Addressing the feelings of unworthiness and getting to the root of them ultimately helps patients follow through with treatment far more effectively than berating them or going over the health benefits again and again. Unless a person feels whole and worthy on the inside, he'll never put in the effort necessary to bring himself back to health.

●-●-●

No matter how poorly a person has followed my instructions, I know it's important that I show them genuine sympathy and congratulate them when they have a success. And that's not difficult for me: when I hear these people's stories, I'm often overwhelmed. I've cried in the office with many of them. Their lives wow me on a daily basis.

That said, I'm not in the business of letting people slide through without any effort or allowing them to rest on their laurels and not keep moving forward. That wouldn't do anyone any good.

Some patients struggle to keep up with the treatment process, but I perceive they are doing the best they can with the resources at their disposal. With this group, we do what they can handle, chipping away at their health problems bit by bit. Other patients, though, are not committed to the healing process, and I think they could do better. These are usually highly intelligent people who have always managed to outsmart their doctors and therapists—they always have a plausible excuse for why they couldn't and shouldn't do something.

When I'm faced with a patient like this, I usually have to be blunt. "You came to me because I treat disease with diet, lifestyle, and supplements, and so far you have been unwilling to change your diet or your lifestyle, or take supplements. So why are you here?"

Once those words are spoken, I don't say another single word until they ask me a question or I have to make an appropriate response. We might sit there in silence for a while, but I don't break eye contact. I just sit back in my chair, eyes open, looking them directly in the face—not staring, but not looking away either.

One time, after about two minutes of silence, the patient stood up and said, "You're being a real prick about this." He stomped out of the room, and I never saw him again. But that's only happened once. Most of the time, people will back up and realize what they need to do to be successful until I see them next. In the more recalcitrant cases, it becomes a series of conversations about their commitment to the plan. Sometimes they'll say, "But I did this and this and this!"

"Well, that's fantastic," I'll say before using my standard line: "You just won the pennant, but we're after the World Series."

Ideally, I'll be able to get these tough, resistant cases to a point where we both understand their deeper, internal obstacles and have found ways to work through them. It's hard work. And in fact, every one of my patients does work hard. No one has it easy.

When people come to me, they're often exhausted, chronically sick, and losing hope. Most aren't thrilled to hear that functional medicine, despite any preconceptions they may have had, is not a magic bullet or a quick fix. They're going to have to work at it, and it's going to take time.

But when the day rolls around that they see firsthand proof of what an incredible tool functional medicine is for overcoming chronic unwellness, I can see on their faces that even the most painful stretches of their journey were one hundred percent worth it.

# AFTERWORD: THE WISDOM PRAYER

*. . . grant me the*

*SERENITY to accept the things I cannot change, the*

*COURAGE to change the things I can, and the*

*WISDOM to know the difference.*

We're often told we live in the information age. But what does that mean? Fundamentally, information is only a sequence of symbols that carries a message. Those messages can be amassed into knowledge—a collection of facts, information, and descriptions pertaining to something or someone.

Wisdom, on the other hand, is a very different thing from both information and knowledge. Wisdom is the judicious application of knowledge. It is a deep understanding of people, things, events, and situations and how they all interrelate. Neither information nor knowledge is adequate in life. One must have wisdom to make impactful, lasting change.

Having courage does not mean you have no fear or that things are easy. In fact, courage is the attribute of making change despite the fact that it is hard or frightening. It is through wisdom and then courage that change is possible.

And what about serenity? Many think of serenity as a passive state, but it's not. Serenity is not the same as surrender. Serenity is an active state, and it starts with forgiveness. One of our most difficult human challenges is to respond to hate or adversity with kindness. We are all touched by heart-warming stories of people who manage to do so, and yet when we confront a life challenge—especially a threat to our health—our default reactions are often anger, angst, depression, anxiety, hate, or any other of many destructive emotions.

Why should we fight against this tendency and strive to forgive? Your enemy, your illness, may not deserve forgiveness, but you do deserve to be free. Holding on to destructive emotions has no positive impact on your illness. Letting go of those emotions and replacing them with love, compassion, and kindness will have a profound effect, whether you're facing a chronic disease or a loved one who's disappointed you. Ancient wisdom tells us that "where love meets adversity, compassion is born."

How do we forgive? We forgive through wisdom. Consider that the Aramaic word for *forgive* means "to untie." We must untie ourselves from the bond of negative emotions surrounding our illness or circumstances. We must understand that the best antidote to illness is to live a happy and successful life, even with our limitations and disabilities. We must seek to find the silver lining in everything, to learn and grow from adversity.

Seek allies on your journey to wellness, among friends, family, and health-care givers. Be compassionate with yourself. So often, our self-talk is destructive. As I advised earlier in this book, speak to yourself like you would speak to your best friend. Use your most compassionate voice. Change your language to reflect a position of strength rather than weakness. In this way, retrain yourself to think not like a passive victim but like an active victor, and maintain perspective. Each of us has an Everest to climb. Each of our Everests is unique.

You may be wondering why I began the Serenity Prayer not with "God" but with ellipses (those three dots). The prayer is often attributed to (but undoubtedly predates) the great theologian Reinhold Niebuhr, and it usually starts with God. Is my replacement disrespectful? I have chosen to use the ellipses because God is bigger than what can be known. Each individual has a concept of God, but each of our concepts is only part of God. *God* is an English word, and many words are used around the world to convey the same meaning. So the use of ellipses is an attempt to enlarge our understanding of a word used to describe the all and the everything. It is an attempt to have each of us pause and think about the word, the world we live in, and what it means to us; after all, what divides us is the petty concern of man. What unites us is the divine concern of God. And whether it's Einstein's God, my God, or your God, it is an *immense* word that demands reflection.

At the core of the Serenity Prayer is one of my fundamental beliefs about being human: that we are uniquely able to exercise control over the fleeting moment in time between stimulus and response. If you apply an electric current to an earthworm, it has no choice but to repel from the stimulus. But we are not earthworms.

A thoughtful, present human being can exercise the full spectrum of human emotion in reacting to a stimulus. When we face something that might normally make us cry, we can stop ourselves and react differently. We can choose to build hope in that moment or maybe even laugh. That requires wisdom.

And how is all of this related to functional medicine? Functional medicine demands much of its practitioners and its patients. Functional medicine attempts to organize the signs, symptoms, and laboratory data into underlying causes. Functional medicine is not just information or knowledge. Functional medicine is the judicious application of knowledge. It is a deep understanding and realization of people, things, events, or situations and how they interrelate. Neither information nor knowledge is adequate; one must have wisdom to make impactful lasting change. This, of course, is the definition of wisdom I first gave. Functional medicine, and the journey you have embarked upon through reading this book, is the relentless pursuit of wisdom.

# ABOUT DR. TOM SULT

Tom Sult is a medical doctor, medical educator, author, and inspirational speaker. Despite all of this education, Tom's early schooling did not go smoothly. By third grade, he was held back and diagnosed with "minimal brain dysfunction," now known as dyslexia. By the end of his second year of third grade, he had been bullied and teased and in school fights nearly every day. It wasn't until the following year that, thanks to a mentor, Tom started understanding that a learning disability (something he now sees as a learning advantage) didn't mean he was stupid.

In high school, another important mentor introduced Tom to the wilderness. He began rock-, snow-, and ice climbing, mountaineering, white water rafting, kayaking, and sailing, and eventually became a guide, calling the mountains his cathedral. Later, Tom supplemented his guiding income with a seven-year stint as a paramedic in emergency rooms and ambulances.

After being rejected from over forty U.S. medical schools (because his grades, due to dyslexia, didn't reflect his knowledge), Tom spent a year in acupuncture school and was then accepted at St. George's University School of Medicine in Grenada, WI. There, he not only attended medical school but also followed and learned from local healers of the "bush doctor" shaman tradition. This experience fit closely with the Eastern traditions he was exposed to in acupuncture school.

After two years in Grenada, Tom transferred to medical school at UCLA, where he was invited to the home of Norman Cousins, a writer and the head of the psychoneuroimmunology department. Over the next two years, Tom spent as much time as possible at the office of psychoneuroimmunology, as he saw it as the scientific embodiment of the Eastern and shamanistic traditions he had experienced in acupuncture school and in Grenada.

The word *doctor* means *teacher*. To Tom, that is the most important definition of what a physician should be. Tom was recognized as the Resident Teacher of the Year as a resident in family medicine and is board-certified in family medicine and integrative holistic medicine. He is on faculty with the

Institute for Functional Medicine, where he has taught hundreds of medical professionals of all disciplines the art of functional medicine. Tom is a contributing author to *The Textbook of Functional Medicine* and other publications and maintains a private practice in Willmar, MN. *Just Be Well* is his first book about functional medicine for the non-medical public.

# APPENDIX A:
# MEDICAL SYMPTOMS QUESTIONNAIRE

This checklist is a catalogue of your current symptoms. The first time you use it, you should be thinking about your general health over the last 30 days. You should then re-evaluate every 30 days, thinking about your general health in the preceding 48 hours to track your progress.

Name _____ Date _____

Rate each of the following symptoms based upon your typical health profile for:

☐ Past 30 days    ☐ Past 48 hours

Point Scale     0  –  Never or almost never have the symptom

                1  –  Occasionally have it, effect is not severe

                2  –  Occasionally have it, effect is severe

                3  –  Frequently have it, effect is not severe

                4  –  Frequently have it, effect is severe


HEAD        _____    Headaches
            _____    Faintness
            _____    Dizziness
            _____    Insomnia                          Total _____


EYES        _____    Watery or itchy eyes
            _____    Swollen, reddened, or sticky eyelids
            _____    Bags or dark circles under eyes
            _____    Blurred or tunnel vision (does not include
                       near- or far-sightedness)          Total _____


EARS        _____    Itchy ears
            _____    Earaches, ear infections
            _____    Drainage from ear
            _____    Ringing in ears, hearing loss       Total _____

0 – Never or almost never have the symptom
1 – Occasionally have it, effect is not severe
2 – Occasionally have it, effect is severe

3 – Frequently have it, effect is not severe
4 – Frequently have it, effect is severe

| | | | |
|---|---|---|---|
| NOSE | _____ | Stuffy nose | |
| | _____ | Sinus problems | |
| | _____ | Hay fever | |
| | _____ | Sneezing attacks | |
| | _____ | Excessive mucus formation | Total _____ |
| | | | |
| MOUTH/ | _____ | Chronic coughing | |
| THROAT | _____ | Gagging, frequent need to clear throat | |
| | _____ | Sore throat, hoarseness, loss of voice | |
| | _____ | Swollen or discolored tongue, gums, lips | |
| | _____ | Canker sores | Total _____ |
| | | | |
| SKIN | _____ | Acne | |
| | _____ | Hives, rashes, dry skin | |
| | _____ | Hair loss | |
| | _____ | Flushing, hot flashes | |
| | _____ | Excessive sweating | Total _____ |
| | | | |
| HEART | _____ | Irregular or skipped heartbeat | |
| | _____ | Rapid or pounding heartbeat | |
| | _____ | Chest pain | Total _____ |
| | | | |
| LUNGS | _____ | Chest congestion | |
| | _____ | Asthma, bronchitis | |
| | _____ | Shortness of breath | |
| | _____ | Difficulty breathing | Total _____ |
| | | | |
| DIGESTIVE | _____ | Nausea, vomiting | |
| TRACT | _____ | Diarrhea | |
| | _____ | Constipation | |
| | _____ | Bloated feeling | |
| | _____ | Belching, passing gas | |
| | _____ | Heartburn | |
| | _____ | Intestinal/stomach pain | Total _____ |

| | | |
|---|---|---|
| JOINTS/ | _____ | Pain or aches in joints |
| MUSCLES | _____ | Arthritis |
| | _____ | Stiffness or limitation of movement |
| | _____ | Pain or aches in muscles |
| | _____ | Feeling of weakness or tiredness |

Total _____

| | | |
|---|---|---|
| WEIGHT | _____ | Binge eating/drinking |
| | _____ | Craving certain foods |
| | _____ | Excessive weight |
| | _____ | Compulsive eating |
| | _____ | Water retention |
| | _____ | Underweight |

Total _____

| | | |
|---|---|---|
| ENERGY/ | _____ | Fatigue, sluggishness |
| ACTIVITY | _____ | Apathy, lethargy |
| | _____ | Hyperactivity |
| | _____ | Restlessness |

Total _____

| | | |
|---|---|---|
| MIND | _____ | Poor memory |
| | _____ | Confusion, poor comprehension |
| | _____ | Poor concentration |
| | _____ | Poor physical coordination |
| | _____ | Difficulty making decisions |
| | _____ | Stuttering or stammering |
| | _____ | Slurred speech |
| | _____ | Learning disabilities |

Total _____

| | | |
|---|---|---|
| EMOTIONS | _____ | Mood swings |
| | _____ | Anxiety, fear, nervousness |
| | _____ | Anger, irritability, aggressiveness |
| | _____ | Depression |

Total _____

| | | |
|---|---|---|
| OTHER | _____ | Frequent illness |
| | _____ | Frequent or urgent urination |
| | _____ | Genital itch or discharge |

Total _____

GRAND TOTAL _____

# APPENDIX B: DISEASE REFERENCE CHART

**SYSTEM IMPLICATED**

| DISEASE | Energy | Assimilation | Bio Transformation | Communication | Defense Repair | Psychological, Social, Spiritual | Structure | Transport |
|---|---|---|---|---|---|---|---|---|
| Acne | | | • | • | | | | |
| ADHD/ADD | | | • | | • | | | |
| Adrenal insufficiency | | | | • | | • | | |
| Allergy | | | | | • | | | |
| Alzheimer's disease | • | | • | | • | | • | |
| Asthma | | | | | • | | | |
| Atrial fibrillation | | | | | | | | • |
| Autoimmune disease | | • | | | • | | | |
| Cancer | • | | • | | • | | | |
| Celiac disease | | • | | | • | | | |
| Chronic fatigue syndrome | • | | • | | • | | • | |
| Coronary artery disease | • | | • | • | • | | | • |
| Dementia | • | | | | • | | • | |
| Dermatitis | | • | • | | • | | | |
| Dermatitis herpetiformis | | • | | | • | | | |
| Diabetes | • | | • | • | • | | | • |
| Endometriosis | | | • | • | | | | |
| Food allergy | | • | | | • | | | |
| Fungal infection, chronic | | | | | • | | | |
| Hypertension | | | | | | | | • |
| Hypochlorhydria | | • | | | | | | |
| Hypogonadism | | | | • | | | | |

| DISEASE | Energy | Assimilation | Bio Transformation | Communication | Defense Repair | Psychological, Social, Spiritual | Structure | Transport |
|---|---|---|---|---|---|---|---|---|
| Hypothyroidism | | | • | • | • | | | |
| Inflammatory bowel disease | | • | • | | • | | | |
| Intestinal permeability (leaky gut) | | • | | | • | | | |
| Irritable bowel syndrome | | • | | | • | | | • |
| Ischemic heart disease | | | | | • | | | • |
| Metabolic syndrome | | | • | • | • | | | • |
| Migraine | • | • | | | | | | |
| Multiple chemical sensitivity | | | • | | • | | | |
| Multiple sclerosis | | | • | | • | | | |
| Nonalcoholic steatohepatitis | | | • | • | • | | | |
| Obesity | • | • | • | • | | | | • |
| Obstructive sleep apnea | | | | | | • | • | |
| Osteoarthritis | | | • | | • | | | |
| Osteoporosis/osteopenia | • | | • | • | | | | |
| Otitis media | | • | | | • | | | |
| Pancreatic insufficiency | | • | | | | | | |
| Parkinson's disease | | | • | | • | | • | |
| Peptic ulcer | | • | | | • | | | |
| Periodontal disease | | | | | • | | | • |
| Polycystic ovary syndrome | | | • | • | | | | |
| Premature ovarian failure | | | • | • | | | | |
| Rheumatoid arthritis | | | • | | • | | | |
| Small bowel bacterial overgrowth | | • | | | | | | |
| Systemic lupus erythematosus | | | • | | • | | | |
| Upper respiratory tract infection, recurrent | | | | | • | | | |
| Urolithiasis | • | | | | | | | |
| Uterine fibroids | | | | • | | | | |

Adapted from *Clinical Pathophysiology: A Functional Perspective: A Systems Approach to Understanding and Reversing Disease Process.*

# APPENDIX C: SYMPTOM REFERENCE CHART

| SYMPTOMS/SIGNS | Energy | Assimilation | Bio Transformation | Communication | Defense Repair | Psychological, Social, Spiritual | Structure | Transport |
|---|---|---|---|---|---|---|---|---|
| Abdominal bloating/gas | | • | | | • | | | |
| Acid-blocking medication | | • | | | • | | | |
| Angina | • | | | | • | | | • |
| Anxiety | | | | • | | • | | |
| Back pain | | | | | • | • | • | |
| Caffeine sensitivity | | | • | | | | | |
| Cognitive function, impaired | • | • | | | | • | • | |
| Common cold, recurrent | | | | | • | | | |
| Constipation | | • | | | | | | |
| Cough, recurrent | | | | | • | | | |
| C-reactive protein, elevated | | | | | • | | | • |
| Dental amalgams, silver | | | • | | | | | |
| Depression | | | • | • | | • | | |
| Diarrhea | | • | | | • | | | |
| Dyslipidemia | | | | • | • | | | • |
| Earache | | | | | • | | | |
| Erectile dysfunction | | | | • | • | | | • |
| Fatigue | • | | | | | • | | • |
| Fingernails, weak, peeling | | • | | | • | | | |
| Fluid retention | | | | • | • | | | • |
| Food hypersensitivity | | • | | | • | | | |
| Gums receding | | | | | • | | • | • |

## SYSTEM IMPLICATED

| SYMPTOMS/SIGNS | Energy | Assimilation | Bio Transformation | Communication | Defense Repair | Psychological, Social, Spiritual | Structure | Transport |
|---|---|---|---|---|---|---|---|---|
| Halitosis | | • | | | | | | |
| Hay fever | • | | | | • | | | |
| Headache | • | | • | • | • | | | |
| Hearing loss | | | | | | | • | |
| Heartburn | | • | | | • | | | |
| Homocysteine, elevated | | | • | | • | | | • |
| Hot flashes | | | • | • | | | | |
| Hyperglycemia | • | | | • | • | | | |
| Indigestion | | • | | | | | | |
| Infertility | | | • | • | | | | |
| Insomnia | | | | | | • | | |
| Insulin resistance | • | | • | • | • | | | • |
| Joint pain | | | • | | • | | • | |
| Learning difficulties | • | • | • | • | • | | | |
| Libido, low | | | | • | | | | |
| Memory loss | • | | • | | | | • | |
| Menopausal symptoms | | | • | • | | | | |
| Menstrual cycle, abnormalities | | | • | • | | | | |
| Muscle weakness | • | | • | | | | • | |
| Premature aging | • | • | • | • | • | | • | |
| Shortness of breath | • | | | | • | | | • |
| Stress, chronic | | | | • | | • | | |
| Urination, frequent | | | • | • | • | | | |
| Urticaria, itching, chronic | | | • | | • | | | |
| Weight gain | | • | • | • | • | | | |
| Wheeze, recurrent | | | • | | • | | | |

Adapted from *Clinical Pathophysiology: A Functional Perspective: A Systems Approach to Understanding and Reversing Disease Process.*

# APPENDIX D: TIMELINE

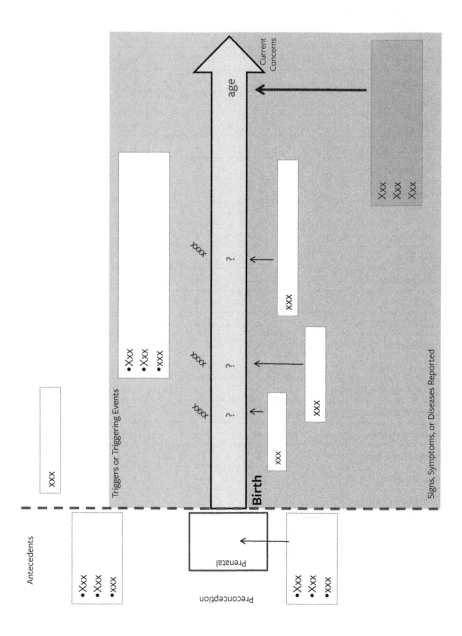

# APPENDIX E: MATRIX

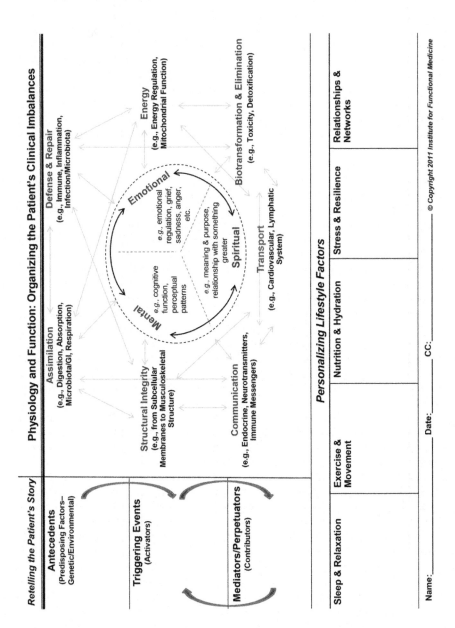

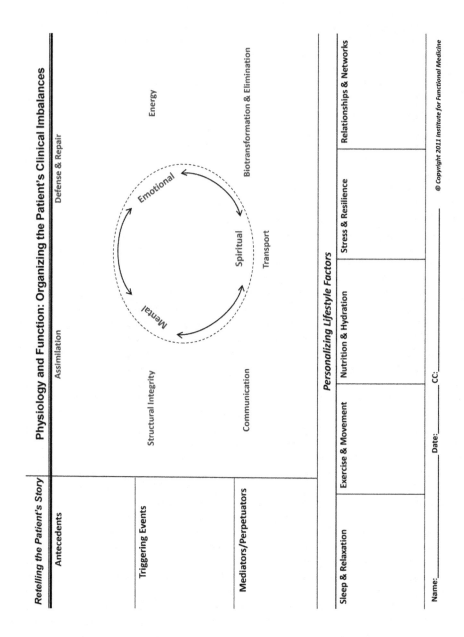

**Physiology and Function: Organizing the Patient's Clinical Imbalances**

*Retelling the Patient's Story*

Antecedents

Triggering Events

Mediators/Perpetuators

Assimilation

Defense & Repair

Energy

Biotransformation & Elimination

Transport

Communication

Structural Integrity

Emotional

Mental

Spiritual

*Personalizing Lifestyle Factors*

| Sleep & Relaxation | Exercise & Movement | Nutrition & Hydration | Stress & Resilience | Relationships & Networks |
|---|---|---|---|---|

Name:_____ Date:_____ CC:_____

© Copyright 2011 Institute for Functional Medicine

# APPENDIX F: FUNCTIONAL MEDICINE CORE PROGRAM

As has already been illustrated, much of defense and repair is actually located in the gut, so optimizing assimilation is almost always an important starting point for regaining wellness. The combination of interventions in the Functional Medicine Core Program is good at eliminating common food sensitivities (diet), reducing inflammation (Ultra-InflamX), reducing dysbiosis (IgG 2000), and improving probiotic activity (ProbioMax). This program also improves phytonutrition and level of antioxidants, and helps with pH balance, oxidative stress (Dynamic Greens), and defense and repair (Dynamic Greens and IgG 2000).

If you're like most of my patients, this program may seem overwhelming at first—particularly the comprehensive elimination diet. But remember, if you can follow at least 90 percent of the rules, you will be well on your way toward regaining *your* dynamic state of well-being.

## COMPREHENSIVE ELIMINATION DIET

The comprehensive elimination diet is a dietary program designed to clear the body of foods and chemicals to which you may be allergic or sensitive. The main rationale behind the diet is that these modifications allow your body's detoxification machinery, which may be overburdened or compromised, to recover and begin to function efficiently again. The dietary changes help the body eliminate or "clear" various toxins that may have accumulated due to environmental exposure, foods, beverages, drugs, alcohol, or cigarette smoking. It also helps reduce inflammation throughout your body.

This is called an "elimination diet" because you remove certain foods, and food categories, from your diet. During a period of six weeks, you eliminate the most likely culprits from your diet. If your symptoms improve during the six-week period, you'll carefully add foods back into your diet one at a time to see which ones may be triggering symptoms. Make sure to read all labels carefully to find hidden allergens. Eat a wide variety of foods, and do not try to restrict your calorie intake. If you find no improvement within six weeks, either you do not have any food allergies, or you may have food allergies, but there is yet another factor complicating the picture. There are no magical answers here; this is a journey of self-exploration and discovery.

I have found this process to be generally well tolerated and extremely beneficial. In fact, it's the best clinical tool I know. There is really no "typical" or "normal" response.

A person's initial response to any new diet is highly variable, and this diet is no exception. This can be attributed to physiological, mental, and biochemical differences among individuals; the degree of exposure to and type of "toxin"; and other lifestyle factors. Most often, individuals on the elimination diet report increased energy and mental alertness, decrease in muscle or joint pain, and a general sense of improved well-being. However, some people report minor initial reactions to the diet, especially in the first week, as their bodies adjust to a different dietary program. Symptoms you may experience in the first week or so can include changes in sleep patterns, lightheadedness, headaches, joint or muscle stiffness, and changes in gastrointestinal function. Such symptoms rarely last more than a few days.

I realize that changing food habits can be a complex, difficult, and sometimes confusing process. It doesn't have to be, and I think that I have simplified the process with diet menus, recipes, snack suggestions, and other information to make it a doable process.

Eat only the foods listed under "Foods to Include," and avoid those foods shown under "Foods to Exclude" in the Comprehensive Elimination Diet Guidelines. These guidelines are intended as a quick overview of the dietary plan. If you have a question about a particular food, check to see if it is on the food list. You should, of course, avoid any listed foods to which you know you are allergic or don't tolerate well. Some of these guidelines may also change based upon your personal health condition and history.

## TIPS

- The first 2–3 days are the hardest. It's important to go shopping to get all of the foods you are allowed to have.

- Plan your meals and have a pot of rice available.

- Eat simply. Cook simply. Make a pot of chicken-vegetable-rice soup. Make a large salad. Cook extra chicken. Have prepared food on hand so you can grab something quickly.

- Eat regular meals.

- You may also want to snack to keep your blood sugar levels normal. It is important to keep blood sugar stable. Carry food with you when you leave the house. That way, you will have what you are allowed and not be tempted to stray off the plan.

- It may be helpful to cook extra chicken, sweet potatoes, rice, beans, etc., that can be reheated for snacking or another meal.

- Avoid any foods that you know or believe you may be sensitive to, even if they are on the "allowed" list.

- Try to eat at least three servings of fresh vegetables each day. Choose at least one serving of dark green or orange vegetables (carrots, broccoli, winter squash) and one raw vegetable each day. Vary your selections.

- This is NOT a weight loss program. If you need to lose or gain weight, work with your practitioner on a program.

- Buy organic produce when possible. Select fresh foods when you can. If possible, choose organically grown fruits and vegetables to eliminate pesticide and chemical residue consumption. Wash fruits and vegetables thoroughly.

- If you are a vegetarian, eliminate the meats and fish, and consume more beans and rice, quinoa, amaranth, teff, millet, and buckwheat.

- If you are consuming coffee or other caffeine-containing beverages on a regular basis, it is always wise to slowly reduce your caffeine intake rather than abruptly stop it; this will prevent caffeine withdrawal headaches. For instance, try drinking half decaf/half regular coffee for a few days, and then slowly reduce the total amount of coffee.

- Read oil labels; use only those that are obtained by a "cold pressed" method.

- If you select animal sources of protein, look for free-range or organically raised chicken, turkey, or lamb. Trim visible fat and prepare by broiling, baking, stewing, grilling, or stir-frying. Cold-water fish (e.g., salmon, mackerel, and halibut) is another excellent source of protein and the omega-3 essential fatty acids, which are important nutrients in this diet. Fish is used extensively.

- Remember to drink the recommended amount (at least two quarts) of plain, filtered water each day.

- Strenuous or prolonged exercise may be reduced during some or the entire program to allow the body to heal more effectively without the additional burden imposed by exercise. Adequate rest and stress reduction is also important to the success of this program.

- You may use leftovers for the next days' meals or part of a meal, e.g., leftover broiled salmon and broccoli from dinner as part of a large salad for lunch the next day.

**Possible Problems:** Most people feel better and better each day during the comprehensive elimination diet. However, if you are used to consuming caffeine, you may get withdrawal symptoms during the first few days, such as headaches, fatigue, irritability, malaise, or increased hunger. If you find your energy lagging, you may need to eat frequently to keep your blood sugar levels (thinking, energy) regular. Be sure to drink plenty of water.

**Testing Individual Foods:** Once you have completed six weeks, you can begin to add foods back into your diet. KEEP A JOURNAL OF ALL FOODS EATEN AND ALL SYMPTOMS. Be sure to add foods one at a time, one every two days. Eat the test food at least twice a day and in a fairly large amount. Often an offending food will provoke symptoms quickly—within 10 minutes to 12 hours. Signs to look for include headache, itching, bloating, nausea, dizziness, fatigue, diarrhea, indigestion, anal itching, sleepiness 30 minutes after a meal, flushing, and/or rapid heartbeat. If you are unsure, take the food back out of your diet for at least one week and try it again. Be sure to test foods in a pure form: for example, test milk or cheese or wheat, but not macaroni and cheese that contains milk, cheese, and wheat!

**The Results:** By avoiding symptom-provoking foods and taking supportive supplements to restore gut integrity, most food allergies/sensitivities will resolve within 4–6 months. This means that in most cases, you will then be able to eat foods that formerly bothered you. In some cases, you will find that the allergy doesn't go away. In this case, either you must wait longer or it may be a "fixed" allergy that will remain lifelong.

**After the Testing:** It would be advisable to return to your health practitioner for a follow-up visit to determine next steps. If you find allergies to many foods, you may want to explore a four-day food rotation diet.

Finally, anytime you change your diet significantly, you may experience such symptoms as fatigue, headache, or muscle aches for a few days. Your body needs time, as it is "withdrawing" from the foods you eat on a daily basis. Your body may crave some foods it is used to consuming. Be patient! Those symptoms generally don't last long, and most people feel much better over the next couple of weeks.

**Enjoy!**

# COMPREHENSIVE ELIMINATION DIET GUIDELINES

| FOODS TO INCLUDE | FOODS TO EXCLUDE |
|---|---|
| **Fruits:** whole fruits, unsweetened, frozen or water-packed, canned fruits, and diluted juices | Oranges and orange juice |
| **Dairy substitutes:** rice milk | **Dairy and eggs:** milk, cheese, eggs, cottage cheese, cream, yogurt, butter, ice cream, frozen yogurt, non-dairy creamers |
| **Non-gluten grains and starch:** rice (all types), millet, quinoa, amaranth, teff, tapioca, buckwheat, potato flour | **Grains:** wheat, corn, barley, spelt, rye, triticale, oat |
| **Animal protein:** fresh or water-packed canned fish, wild game, lamb, duck, organic chicken and turkey | Pork, beef/veal, sausage, cold cuts, canned meats, frankfurters, shellfish |
| **Vegetable protein:** split peas, lentils, and legumes | Soybean products (soy sauce, soybean oil in processed foods; tempeh, tofu, soy milk, soy yogurt, textured vegetable protein) |
| **Nuts and seeds:** coconut, pine nuts, flax seeds | Peanuts and peanut butter; walnuts; sesame, pumpkin, and sunflower seeds; hazelnuts; pecans; almonds; cashews; nut butters such as almond or tarini |
| **Vegetables:** all raw, steamed, sautéed, juiced, or roasted vegetables | Corn, creamed vegetables. If you have arthritis, avoid nightshades: tomatoes, potatoes, eggplants, peppers, paprika, salsa, chili peppers, cayenne, chili powder. |
| **Oils:** cold-pressed olive, ghee | Butter, margarine, shortening, processed oils, salad dressings, mayonnaise (and similar spreads), flax, safflower, sesame, almond, sunflower, walnut, canola, pumpkin |
| **Drinks:** filtered or distilled water, decaffeinated herbal teas, seltzer or mineral water | Alcohol, coffee, and other caffeinated beverages; soda pop or soft drinks |
| **Sweeteners (use sparingly):** brown rice syrup, agave nectar, stevia, fruit sweetener, blackstrap molasses | Refined sugar, white/brown sugars, honey, maple syrup, high fructose corn syrup, evaporated cane juice |
| **Condiments:** vinegar; all spices, including salt, pepper, basil, carob, cinnamon, cumin, dill, garlic, ginger, mustard, oregano, parsley, rosemary, tarragon, thyme, turmeric | Chocolate, ketchup, relish, chutney, soy sauce, barbecue sauce, teriyaki, and other condiments |

## THINGS TO WATCH FOR:

- Corn starch in baking powder and any processed foods
- Corn syrup in beverages and processed foods
- Vinegar in ketchup, mayonnaise, and mustard is usually from wheat or corn.
- Breads advertised as gluten-free, which contain oats, spelt, Kamut (khorasan wheat), rye
- Many amaranth and millet flake cereals have oats or corn.
- Many canned tunas contain textured vegetable protein, which is from soy; look for low-salt versions, which tend to be pure tuna with no fillers.

READ ALL INGREDIENT LABELS CAREFULLY

## MENU IDEAS

Here are some ideas to stimulate your creativity. Feel free to invent your own recipes and menus. Items marked with an asterisk (*) indicate that a recipe follows.

### BREAKFAST

Feel free to add protein powder drinks, leftover chicken, fish, etc., to your breakfast menu.

- Cooked whole grain (oatmeal, cream of brown rice, buckwheat, teff, millet, or quinoa) served with fresh or frozen fruit. Can add a bit of coconut, ghee, sweetener, and/or cinnamon. To boost protein, have a rice protein powder drink.

- Home fried potatoes: Cut onions, peppers, broccoli, mushrooms, and other vegetables of your choice into small pieces and sauté in olive oil or ghee. Cut pre-baked potatoes into cubes and add to vegetables. Add salt, pepper, herbs, and/or spices.

- "Fried" rice: Use recipe above. Add rice instead of potatoes.

- Toasted rice or lentil flax bread, with coconut oil or ghee, 100% fruit jam or apple or pear butter, fresh fruit, herbal tea.

- Fruit smoothie: Blend rice milk with fruit. Possible additions: berries, bananas, pears, pineapple, mango, papaya, etc. Add flax seeds or psyllium seeds as desired. Add fish oil as desired. Eat on its own or as part of a breakfast.

- Rice pancakes* topped with apple butter, applesauce, or sautéed apples.

- Cole rice or amaranth or other gluten-free cereal (read label carefully) with fresh fruit (bananas, berries, pears, apples, etc.) and rice milk.

- Sweet potato delight*, half a cantaloupe filled with blueberries or half a papaya with lime juice.

- Mochi rice waffles* topped with sautéed apples*; fruit smoothie with rice protein powder.

- Breakfast rice pudding*, rice milk, berries.

### LUNCH OR DINNER

- Large salad with grilled chicken or fish. Serve with gluten-free bread or baked potato, baked winter squash, or boiled new potatoes.

- Broiled salmon plus steamed or oven-roasted vegetables with cooked millet or baked potato, baked sweet potato, or quinoa salad. Can also add a salad with vinaigrette dressing.

- Asparagus soup* (or other soup), cabbage salad*, rice cakes with ghee, fresh fruit.

- Broiled lamb chop, green rice*, cooked vegetables, fruity spinach salad*.

- Fruit salad with coconut or pine nuts served with protein and rice crackers.

- Broiled or poached halibut, baked winter squash sprinkled with cinnamon and ghee, mixed green salad with vinaigrette dressing, and mochi rice squares and fruit for dessert.

- Brown rice and grilled chicken, steamed greens, baked potato or sweet potato.

- Halibut salad: mixed greens of your choice, leftover halibut cut into chunks, vinaigrette dressing. Serve with baked potato with ghee.

- Chicken breast sprinkled with garlic powder and tarragon, steamed asparagus or broccoli, brown or wild rice or kasha, ghee or olive oil.

- Quinoa with chicken vegetable soup or vegetable soup.

- Quinoa salad with leftover chicken or fish.

- Chicken salad: leftover chicken, mixed greens, guacamole, millet with pine nuts.

- Fresh tuna steak topped with herbs and broiled, rice pasta with olive oil and mock pesto*, steamed kale or collard greens tossed with olive oil and garlic and vinegar, mixed green salad with vinaigrette dressing. Fruit for dessert.

- Tuna salad: canned tuna mixed with vinaigrette or eggless mayonnaise, baking powder biscuits*, fresh fruit.

- Roast turkey breast or broiled turkey burger, brown or wild rice, steamed vegetable, salad with vinaigrette. Baked apple or poached pear.

- Turkey salad: leftover turkey breast, mixed greens, other fresh vegetables, lemon or oil and vinegar, rice crackers or baking powder biscuits*, fresh fruit or cup of soup.

- Rice pasta primavera*, pickled beets*, mixed green salad with vinaigrette, leftover breakfast rice pudding topped with berries.

## SNACKS

- Rice cakes or crackers with ghee, unsweetened apple butter, or coconut oil; raw carrot

- Guacamole* on rice cakes

- Vegetables dipped into guacamole

- Baked apple

- Poached pear*

- Bowl of soup and rice crackers

- Rice cakes or crackers spread with apple butter

- Fresh fruit

- Fresh vegetables: carrots, cucumbers, sweet peppers, etc.

- Mochi rice squares, plain or with apple butter or smashed berries

- Baked sweet potatoes

# RECIPES

## BREAKFAST

### Breakfast Rice Pudding • *Serves 4*

1 cup uncooked short grain brown rice
1¼ cups coconut milk
1¼ cups water

½ tsp. salt
1 Tbsp. brown rice syrup
1 tsp. cinnamon

Combine water and coconut milk in heavy pot; bring to boil, adding rice and salt. Simmer, covered (do NOT stir) for about 45 minutes or more, until liquid is mostly absorbed and rice is soft. Remove from heat and allow to cool for 15 minutes. Stir in brown rice syrup and cinnamon.

### Mochi Rice Waffles • *Serves 4*

Purchase 1 package of cinnamon-apple mochi and defrost.
Cut into quarters. Slice each quarter across to form 2 thinner squares.
Place one square into preheated waffle iron and cook until done.
Top with your choice of fruit or sautéed apples (*below*).

### Rice Pancakes • *Makes approximately 14 (4-inch) pancakes*

1⅓ cups rice flour
½ cup millet flour
2 tsp. baking powder
½ tsp. baking soda
¼ tsp. salt

1 Tbsp. apple butter
1 Tbsp. ghee
Egg replacer to equal 2 eggs (*refer to recipe below*)
1½ cups rice milk
1½ Tbsp. apple cider vinegar

Mix the almond or rice milk with the vinegar and allow mixture to stand for 5 minutes until curdles form. Mix dry ingredients together and set aside. In large mixing bowl, beat apple butter, oil, egg, and milk. Add dry mixture and stir gently. Be careful not to over mix. Serve with sautéed apples (*refer to recipe below*).

### Sweet Potato Delight • *Serves 1–2*

1 ripe banana
1 medium sweet potato, cooked
1 tsp. oil

1 Tbsp. fruit sweetener, molasses, or
brown rice syrup (optional)

Shake the pan often. Cut the banana in half lengthwise. Cut the cooked sweet potato into ½″ pieces. Add the oil to the pan. Place the banana pieces, flat sides down, in the pan. Add the sweet potatoes. Cover and cook for 2 minutes. Uncover, and cook for 5 minutes until everything is heated through and browned on one side. Add the sweetener before serving.

Adapted and used with permission from *The Allergy Self Help Cookbook* by Marjorie Hurt Jones, R.N. Rodale Press, Emmaus, PA.

**Oven-Roasted Veggies** • *Number of servings depends on amount of veggies used*

Use any combination of the following vegetables, unpeeled, washed, and cut into bite-sized pieces: eggplant, small red potatoes, red onion, yellow or green summer squash, mushrooms, asparagus. Toss with crushed garlic cloves and olive oil, and sprinkle with rosemary, oregano, tarragon, and basil to taste. Spread in roasting pan in single layers and roast approximately 20–25 minutes at 400 degrees until veggies are tender and slightly brown, stirring occasionally. The amount of time needed depends on the size of the veggie. Salt and pepper to taste. Serve while warm, or use cold leftovers in salad.

**Mock Pesto** • *Makes 1 cup*

1 large ripe avocado
1 cup basil leaves
¼ tsp. lemon juice
¼ cup pine nuts

1 garlic clove, minced or ⅛ tsp. garlic
  powder
½ tsp. olive or flax oil

Cut the avocado in half and remove the pit. Scoop out the flesh and place it in the bowl of a food processor. Add the basil, garlic, and pine nuts. Process for about 2 minutes, scraping the bowl as necessary. Transfer it to a small bowl and coat the surface with oil to prevent browning. Chill.

Used with permission from *The Allergy Self Help Cookbook* by Marjorie Hurt Jones, R.N. Rodale Press, Emmaus, PA.

**Rice Pasta Primavera** • *Serves 4*

2 cups uncooked rice pasta (noodles,
  spaghetti, or elbows)
1 large whole chicken breast, cut into
  thin strips (optional)
Broccoli florets, chopped carrot, and/or
  other favorite veggie, lightly steamed

3–4 scallions, chopped
2 cloves garlic, minced
1 Tbsp. olive oil (more if needed)
¼ cup fresh basil, finely chopped
¼ to ½ cup coconut milk

Cook rice pasta according to package directions. While pasta is cooking, heat oil in wok or heavy frying pan, and stir fry chicken strips or tofu chunks, garlic, scallions, and basil for about 5 minutes. Add remaining vegetables and coconut milk and continue to cook until veggies are soft and glisten. Add more coconut milk as needed. Remove from heat, spoon over drained rice pasta, and garnish with black olives and extra olive oil, if desired.

## SOUPS AND STOCK

### Asparagus Soup • *Serves 4*

1 lb. asparagus, trimmed
2 medium leeks or 4 large shallots
1 Tbsp. oil
2–3 cloves garlic, minced

2 cups water or chicken stock
1 tsp. dried dill weed
Pinch of nutmeg

Slice off the tips of the asparagus and reserve them. Cut the remaining stalks into 1″ pieces. Slice the leeks in half lengthwise and wash under cold water to remove any sand. Slice into ¼″ pieces. Sauté the leeks or shallots in the oil over medium heat until soft. Add the garlic and sliced asparagus stalks. Cook, stirring, another minute or two. Add the water or stock and dill. Simmer 10–12 minutes.

Remove from heat, allow to cool 5–10 minutes. Puree half the volume at a time. Return to pan, add the reserved asparagus tips, and simmer 3–5 minutes or until tips are just barely tender. Add nutmeg. If soup is too thick, thin with additional water or stock.

Used with permission from *The Allergy Self Help Cookbook* by Marjorie Hurt Jones, R.N. Rodale Press, Emmaus, PA.

### Basic Stock Recipe

In a stockpot, put 2 pounds bones, skin, and cartilage from poultry, fish, beef, lamb, or shellfish. (If you use a whole chicken, cook for about an hour; then take meat off the bones. Toss bones and connective tissue back into the pot. Leave the meat aside.)

Cover with water (2–3 quarts) and add:

1–2 Tbsp. of lemon juice or vinegar
1–2 tsp. salt
½ tsp. pepper

Carrots, onions, celery
Parsley, sage, rosemary, thyme, bay

Cook several hours (4–24) on low temperature or in a crock pot. Skim off scum/solids from top of soup after a couple of hours. Remove bones. Skim off fat. (Sometimes it is easiest to refrigerate and then skim off fat.) Either strain and use as broth or begin adding vegetables, grains, etc., to make a soup. Can be used to cook grains or vegetables instead of water.

### Beef Stock

About 4 lbs. beef marrow and knuckle
  bones
1 calf's foot, cut into pieces (optional)
3 lbs. meaty rib or neck bones
4 or more quarts cold filtered water
½ cup vinegar
3 onions, coarsely chopped

3 carrots, coarsely chopped
3 celery stalks, coarsely chopped
Several sprigs of fresh thyme, tied
  together
1 teaspoon dried green peppercorns,
  crushed
1 bunch parsley

Place the knuckle and marrow bones (and optional calf's foot) in a very large pot with vinegar and cover with water. Let stand for one hour. Meanwhile, place the meaty bones in a roasting pan and brown at 350 degrees in the oven. When well browned, add to the pot along with the vegetables. Pour the fat out of the roasting pan, add cold water to the pan, set over a high flame, and bring to a boil, stirring with a wooden spoon to loosen up coagulated juices. Add this liquid to the pot. Add additional water, if necessary, to cover the bones, but the liquid should come no higher than within one inch of the rim of the pot, as the volume expands slightly during cooking. Bring to a boil. A large amount of scum will come to the top, and it is important to remove this with a spoon. After you have skimmed, reduce heat and add the thyme and crushed peppercorns.

Simmer stock for at least 12 hours and as long as 72 hours. Just before finishing, add the parsley and simmer another 10 minutes. You will now have a pot of rather repulsive-looking brown liquid containing globs of gelatinous and fatty material. It doesn't even smell particularly good. But don't despair. After straining it, you will have a delicious and nourishing clear broth that forms the basis for many other recipes in this book.

Remove bones with tongs or a slotted spoon. Strain the stock into a large bowl. Let cool in the refrigerator and remove the congealed fat that rises to the top. Transfer to smaller containers and place in the freezer for long-term storage.

Recipe courtesy of Sally Fallon, *Nourishing Traditions.*

## SALADS AND VEGETABLES

### Cabbage Salad • *Serves 4–6*

1 small to medium head red cabbage, thinly sliced (or use half red and half green cabbage)
8 sliced radishes or 1 grated carrot
3 green apples, diced

1 stalk celery, chopped
Dash of garlic powder
2 Tbsp. olive oil
2 tsp. vinegar
1 tsp. lemon juice

Mix all ingredients in a bowl and allow to sit for one hour, stirring once or twice. Serve cold or at room temperature.

### Fruity Spinach Salad • *Serves 6–8*

1 lb. fresh spinach, washed, dried, torn into pieces

1 pint fresh organic strawberries or raspberries, washed

Dressing:
3 Tbsp. pine nuts
2 scallions, chopped

½ cup olive or flax oil
¼ cup balsamic vinegar

Cut berries in half and arrange over spinach in serving bowl. Combine dressing ingredients in blender or food processor and process until smooth. Just before serving, pour over salad and toss. Garnish with nuts.

## Guacamole • *Makes 1½–2 cups*

2–3 ripe avocados
¼ cup chopped onions
¼ tsp. vitamin C crystals

1 Tbsp. water
1 small clove garlic, chopped

Cut the avocados in half, remove the pits, and scoop the flesh into a blender or food processor. Add the onions, vitamin C crystals, water, and garlic. Process until smooth. Transfer to a small bowl. Cover and chill. Use within 2–3 days. To prevent darkening, coat top with a thin layer of oil. For a chunky version, mash the avocado with a fork and finely chop onions and garlic.

Used with permission from *The Allergy Self Help Cookbook* by Marjorie Hurt Jones, R.N. Rodale Press, Emmaus, PA.

## Pickled Beets • *Serves 4–6*

4 beets, cooked and skinned
¼ cup water
1 Tbsp. brown rice syrup or fruit sweetener

¼ cup rice vinegar
¼ tsp. ground cinnamon
Pinch each of cloves and allspice

Combine the water, sweetener, vinegar, cinnamon, cloves, and allspice in a medium saucepan. Simmer for 2 minutes. Stir in the beets, and heat through. Serve hot or warm.

Adapted with permission from *The Allergy Self Help Cookbook* by Marjorie Hurt Jones, R.N. Rodale Press, Emmaus, PA.

## Quinoa Salad • *Serves 8–10*

1½ cups quinoa, rinsed several times
3 cups water, or chicken broth or vegetable broth (or a combination)
1 cup fresh or frozen peas (frozen baby peas should be just defrosted)
Chopped veggies, raw or lightly steamed (broccoli, asparagus, green beans, etc.)
½ cup chopped red onion

1 pint cherry tomatoes (optional)
½ cup chopped black olives (optional)
⅓ cup olive oil
2 Tbsp. balsamic vinegar or lemon juice
1 or 2 crushed garlic cloves
2–4 Tbsp. fresh dill, chopped (or 1 Tbsp. dried dill)
2 Tbsp. chopped fresh parsley
Salt and pepper to taste

Rinse quinoa well (quinoa tastes bitter if not well rinsed). Bring 3 cups water or broth to a boil. Add rinsed quinoa and bring back to boil. Simmer uncovered for about 15 minutes until liquid is well absorbed. Transfer to large bowl with a small amount of olive oil to prevent sticking, and allow to cool. Meantime, mix together remaining oil, vinegar or lemon juice, parsley, and garlic in a small bowl. Add veggies to quinoa and toss well with dressing mixture, dill, salt, and pepper. Chill before serving.

**Vinaigrette Dressing** • *6 servings* (*approximately*)

*Note: ingredient amounts in this recipe are approximate—use more or less of certain ingredients to adapt recipe to your personal taste.*

½ cup extra virgin olive oil

3 Tbsp. balsamic vinegar (preferred because it has the richest flavor)

2–3 Tbsp. water

1 tsp. dry mustard

1–3 cloves fresh garlic (whole pieces for flavor or crushed for stronger taste)

Salt and pepper to taste

Oregano, basil, parsley, tarragon, or any herbs of your choice, fresh or dried

Place vinegar, water, and mustard in a tightly capped jar, and shake well to thoroughly dissolve mustard. Add oil and remaining ingredients; shake well again. Store refrigerated and shake well before using. Dressing will harden when cold; allow 5–10 minutes to re-liquify.

## GRAINS/BREADS

**Basic Kasha** • *Serves 4–5*

1 cup buckwheat groats

2 cups water, or chicken or vegetable broth

Roast the dry buckwheat groats over medium heat in a dry skillet, stirring until the grains begin to smell toasty, about 2 minutes. Add the water or broth, cover, and simmer for 20–30 minutes, until kasha is tender but not mushy. Pour off any excess liquid.

Optional: add onion, garlic, and herbs to the dish.

**Baking Powder Biscuits** • *Makes one dozen*

1½ cups brown rice flour

½ cup tapioca flour

4 tsp. baking powder

⅛ tsp. salt

3 Tbsp. ghee

1 cup applesauce, unsweetened

Preheat oven to 425 degrees. In a medium-large mixing bowl, stir together dry ingredients. Sprinkle oil on top and mix well with a pastry blender or fork until consistency is crumbly. Mix in applesauce and stir until blended. Spoon heaping tablespoonfuls onto ungreased cookie sheet. With spoon, lightly shape into biscuit. Bake 15–18 minutes until slightly browned. Serve warm for best flavor, but may be lightly reheated in a microwave.

**Green Rice** • *Serves 4*

1 cup brown basmati rice
2 cups water
¼ to ½ tsp. salt
1 bunch parsley
1 clove garlic

1½ Tbsp. lemon juice
1½ Tbsp. olive oil
½ cucumber, diced
Pepper to taste

Bring water to a boil, add rice and salt, stir and simmer, covered, for 45 minutes. Remove from heat and let sit for another 10 minutes. Remove cover and allow to cool. While rice is cooking, blend almonds, parsley, garlic, and oil in a food processor. When rice is cool, stir with nut mixture and add pepper to taste. Garnish with cucumber if desired.

**Meal in a Muffin** • *Makes one dozen*

1 medium carrot, grated
1 large apple, grated
¼ cup ghee
¼ cup unsweetened applesauce
Egg replacement to equal 2 eggs
⅓ cup rice syrup, molasses, or agave
  (or mixture of those sweeteners)
2 tsp. vanilla

¼ cup millet flour
½ cup brown rice flour
¼ tsp. cinnamon
½ tsp. baking powder
¼ tsp. ginger
⅛ tsp. nutmeg
¼ cup shredded unsweetened coconut
½ cup dates

Preheat oven to 375 degrees. Mix all wet ingredients and set aside. In a separate bowl, mix dry ingredients and then mix both together. Lightly coat muffin tins with oil spray. Fill ¾ full and bake 15–20 minutes or until toothpick comes out clean. Allow to cool on a rack.

Adapted with permission from *Wheat-free Sugar-Free Gourmet Cooking* by Sue O'Brien, Gig Harbor, WA, 2001.

**Yellow Rice**

2 cups chicken stock
1 small onion, finely chopped
2 tsp. olive oil

1 clove garlic, minced
½ tsp. turmeric
1 cup uncooked long grain brown rice

In a 2-quart saucepan over low heat, sauté onions in oil until tender, about 5 minutes. Add the garlic and sauté 1 minute. Stir in turmeric, then rice. Add stock. Bring to a boil, cover and simmer 45 minutes over low heat, or until rice is tender and liquid is absorbed. Do not stir. Spoon beans over rice.

# FRUIT

## Baked Apple • *Serves 6*

⅓ cup golden raisins
2 Tbsp. apple juice
6 cooking apples, cored
1½ cups water
2 tsp. pure vanilla extract

¼ cup frozen unsweetened apple juice
concentrate
1 tsp. cinnamon
1 tsp. arrowroot

Remove peel from top third of each apple and arrange in a small baking dish. In a medium saucepan, combine other ingredients and bring to a boil, stirring frequently. Reduce heat and simmer 2–3 minutes, until slightly thickened. Distribute raisins, filling centers of each apple. Pour sauce over apples and bake, uncovered, at 350 degrees for 1 to 1½ hours. Baste occasionally and remove from oven when apples are pierced easily with a fork. Spoon juice over apples and serve warm.

## Poached Pears • *Serves 6*

6 pears
2" stick cinnamon or 1 tsp. cinnamon
1 tsp. cardamom

2 cups apple juice or apple cranberry
juice

Peel pears or leave whole. Place in covered casserole dish in oven or soup pot on stove. Cook until soft, about 30–60 minutes depending on the ripeness of the pears.

## Sautéed Apples • *Serves 2*

2 apples, washed
½ Tbsp. olive oil or ghee

2 tsp. cinnamon
2–3 Tbsp. apple juice

Thinly slice apples and sauté in oil until softened. Add cinnamon and apple juice and simmer, stirring, uncovered for a few more minutes.

# MISCELLANEOUS

## Corn-Free Baking Powder

2 tsp. cream of tartar
2 tsp. arrowroot

1 tsp. baking soda

Sift together to mix well. Store in an airtight container. Make small batches.

**Egg Replacer** • *Equals one egg*

⅓ cup water                                    1 Tbsp. whole or ground flaxseed

Place the water and flaxseed together and allow to gel for about 5 minutes. This mixture will bind patties, meat loaves, cookies, and cakes as well as eggs do, but it will not leaven like eggs for soufflés or sponge cakes. Increase amounts accordingly for additional egg replacement.

**Nutty Mayo** • *Makes 1¼ cups (keeps well for 3 weeks)*

½ cup pine nuts                              1 Tbsp. brown rice syrup
¾ cup water                                   1 Tbsp. minced parsley
3 Tbsp. vinegar                              1 Tbsp. snipped chives
2 Tbsp. oil                                      1½ tsp. dry mustard
1 Tbsp. arrowroot

Grind the pine nuts to a fine powder in a blender. Add the water, blend 1 minute to make sure the pine nuts are fully ground. Add the vinegar, oil, arrowroot, sweetener, and seasonings. Blend until very smooth. Pour into a saucepan and cook a few minutes, until thick. Allow to cool, transfer to a glass jar. Store in the refrigerator.

Adapted and used with permission from *The Allergy Self Help Cookbook* by Marjorie Hurt Jones, R.N. Rodale Press, Emmaus, PA.

# SHOPPING LIST

## The Comprehensive Elimination Diet

### Fats & Oils

Servings / day ______ □□□□□□□□□

2 T.....Avocado
1½ T..Coconut milk (⅓ c light)
8........Olives, black or green
1 t......Oils, cooking or unrefined: Coconut (virgin), Olive (extra virgin), Ghee
1 T.....Pesto (Olive oil, cheese free)

*1 serving = 45 calories, 5 g fat*

**ELIMINATE**

| | | | |
|---|---|---|---|
| Butter | Salad dressings | Canola | Sesame |
| Margarine | Shortening | Grapeseed | Soybean |
| Mayonnaise | **Oils:** | Pumpkin | Sunflower |
| Processed oils | Almond | Safflower | Walnut |

### Nuts & Seeds

Servings / day ______ □□□□□□□□□

3 T.....Coconut (unsweetened)
2 T.....Flax seed, ground
1 T.....Pine nuts

*1 serving = 45 calories, 5 g fat*

**ELIMINATE**

| | | | |
|---|---|---|---|
| Almonds | Hazelnuts | Pistachios | Sunflower seeds |
| Brazil nuts | Peanuts | Pumpkin seeds | Walnuts |
| Cashews | Pecans | Sesame | Nut butters |

### Protein

Servings / day ______ □□□□□□□□□

**Plant Protein:** (*organic, non GMO preferred*)
1 oz...Burger alternatives: mushroom, veggie, no soy
**Animal Proteins (very lean cuts or organic)**
1 oz...Fish (fresh, frozen, wild-caught, not farm raised)
1 oz...Meat: buffalo, elk, lamb, venison, wild game
1 oz...Poultry (skinless chicken, turkey, Cornish hen)
2sm...Sardines
1 oz...Seafood, no shell fish
**Protein Powder:**
Check label for #grams/scoop (1 protein serving = 7 g)
Rice, pea, hemp protein, no soy, whey, or egg white

*1 oz serving = 50-100 calories, 7 g pro*

**ELIMINATE**

| | | | |
|---|---|---|---|
| Beef/veal | Frankfurters | **Soy:** | Nato |
| Canned meats | Pork | Tofu | TVP |
| Cold cuts | Sausage | Tempe | |
| Eggs | Shellfish | Miso | |

### Non-starchy Vegetables

Servings / day ______ ■■■■■■■■

| | | |
|---|---|---|
| Artichoke | Celery | Mushrooms (Crimini Shiitake) |
| Asparagus | Chard/Swiss Chard | Okra |
| Bamboo shoots | Cucumbers | Onions |
| Bean sprouts | Greens (beet, dandelion, collard, kale, mustard, turnip) | Radish |
| Bell peppers | Green beans | Shallots |
| Bok choy | Jicama | Spinach |
| Broccoli | Leeks | Squash, summer |
| Brussels sprouts | Lettuce | Vegetable juice (¾ c) |
| Cabbage | | Fermented vegetables (kimchi, sauerkraut) |
| Carrots | | |
| Cauliflower | | |

*1 serving = ½ c cooked, 1 c raw, 10- 25 calories, 5 g carb*

**Avoid the following as directed by your healthcare provider:**

| | | | |
|---|---|---|---|
| Cayenne | Eggplant | Peppers (bell, chili, hot) | Tomatillo |
| Chili powder | Paprika | Pimento | Salsa |
| Tomato | | | |

### Legumes

Servings / day ______ ■■■■■■■■

½ c....Cooked dried peas, beans, or lentils
¾ c....Bean soups
⅓ c....Hummus or other bean dips
½ c....Fat-free refried beans

*1 serving = 110 calories, 15 g carb, 7 g pro*

**ELIMINATE (if not vegetarian)**

Soybean products (soy sauce, soybean oil in processed foods; tempeh, tofu, soy milk, soy yogurt, textured vegetable protein)

### Low-fat Dairy/ Alternatives

Servings / day ______ ■■■■■■■■

8 oz...Milk alternatives: rice, coconut
*8 oz...Dairy-free coconut yogurt or kiefer*
2 oz...Vegan style rice milk cheeses

*1 serving = 70-100 calories, 12 g carb, 7 g pro*

**ELIMINATE**

| | | |
|---|---|---|
| Butter | Frozen yogurt | Milk alternatives: nut, hemp, soy |
| Cheese | Ice cream | Yogurt |
| Cottage cheese | Milk | Non-dairy creamers |
| Cream | | |

### Starchy Vegetables

Servings / day ______ ■■■■■■■■

1 c.....Acorn squash, cubed
1 c.....Beets, cubed
1 c.....Butternut squash, cubed
½ c....Green peas
⅓ c....Plantain (½ whole)
1 c.....Snow peas
½md .Potato, white
½ c....Potato, white (mashed)
½ c...Winter roots or squashes, (acorn, beet, butternut, parsnip, pumpkin, turnip)

*1 serving = 80 calories, 15 g carb*

**ELIMINATE**

| | |
|---|---|
| Corn | Potato (if avoiding nightshades) |

### Fruits (No sugar added)

Servings / day ______ ■■■■■■■■

| | | |
|---|---|---|
| 1 sm .Apple | ½ c....Fruit juice | 2 sm..Plums |
| ½ c....Applesauce (unsweetened) | 15......Grape | 1 sm..Pomegranate |
| 4........Apricots, fresh | ½ sm.Mango | 3 md .Prunes |
| ½.......Banana, med | 1 c.....Melon | 2 T.....Raisins |
| ¾ c....Blackberries | 1 sm..Nectarine | 1 c.....Raspberries |
| ¾ c....Blueberries | 1 c.....Papaya | 2 sm..Tangerines |
| 12......Cherries | 1 sm..Peach | 2 T.....Dried fruit |
| 3........Dates or Figs | 1 sm..Pear | |
| | ¾ c....Pineapple | |

*1 serving = 60 calories, 15 g carb*

**ELIMINATE**

| | |
|---|---|
| Oranges | Orange juice |

### Grains

Servings / day ______ ■■■■■■■■

| | | |
|---|---|---|
| Amaranth* | Potato flour* | Sorghum* |
| Basmati rice* | Quinoa* | Tapioca* |
| Buckwheat/kasha* | Rice* | Teff* |
| Millet* | | |

*Serving = ⅓-½ c*

½ c....Cereal, cooked (rice)
¾ c....Cereal, ready-to-eat (rice)
⅓ c....Quinoa*
⅓ c....Rice*
1 sl. ...Rice bread*
2 .......Rice cakes (brown)*
3-4.....Rice crackers*
⅓ c....Rice noodles or pasta*

** = Gluten free*

*1 serving = 75-110 calories, 15 g carb*

**ELIMINATE**

| | | | |
|---|---|---|---|
| Barley | Oat | Spelt | Wheat |
| Corn | Rye | Triticale | |

* all measurements in single serving sizes

© 2012 The Institute for Functional Medicine

After six weeks of following the comprehensive elimination diet, refer to your medical symptoms questionnaire and evaluate which symptoms have reduced in frequency and/or intensity.

Generally, 70% of people will feel 50% better at this point in the program. Unfortunately, the second 50% comes a little harder. Now is when you should begin reintroducing one new food at a time. When you find a healthy food that agrees with you (causing no symptoms), you can safely add it to your diet. If you discover a food that disagrees with you, leave it out for three months before retrying. During this reintroduction process, keep all supplements (refer to page 208) constant. You should keep a journal of how you feel during this reintroduction. During this time, you will likely need the support and expertise of a functional medicine doctor.

If you saw no improvement in the first six weeks, you should definitely visit a practitioner of functional medicine for a deeper look. (As Abraham Lincoln said, "A person who represents himself has a fool for a client!")

In order to prevent you from falling back into old habits, now is the time to start transitioning from the elimination diet to what I call the core diet. The core diet is a healthy, low glycemic index, high fruit and vegetable eating program. It is designed to be your long-term lifestyle choice. What follows is an explanation of the core diet plan (1,600 calories for women and 2,000 calories for men) along with some specific food suggestions.

# CORE DIET, 1,600 CALORIES

## CORE FOOD PLAN

### DAILY FOOD INTAKE

### DAILY FLUID INTAKE

% of your desirable weight (lbs) in ounces

**Best Choice:** Purified water

**Other Options:**
Unsweetened beverages low in salt/sodium and caffeine

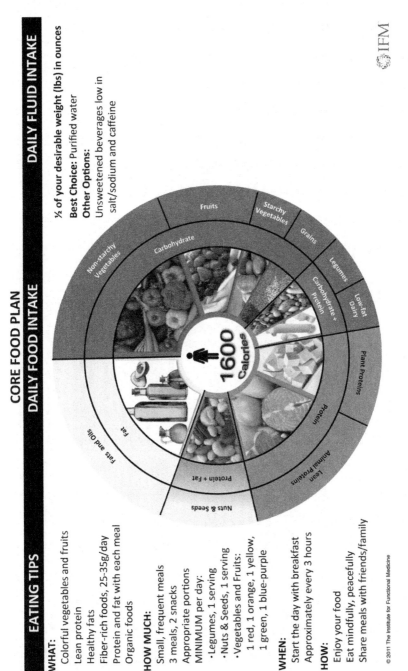

### EATING TIPS

**WHAT:**
Colorful vegetables and fruits
Lean protein
Healthy fats
Fiber-rich foods, 25-35g/day
Protein and fat with each meal
Organic foods

**HOW MUCH:**
Small, frequent meals
3 meals, 2 snacks
Appropriate portions
MINIMUM per day:
• Legumes, 1 serving
• Nuts & Seeds, 1 serving
• Vegetables and Fruits:
1 red, 1 orange, 1 yellow,
1 green, 1 blue-purple

**WHEN:**
Start the day with breakfast
Approximately every 3 hours

**HOW:**
Enjoy your food
Eat mindfully, peacefully
Share meals with friends/family

© 2011 The Institute for Functional Medicine

# Fats & Oils

**6** Servings / day □□□□□□

| | | | |
|---|---|---|---|
| 2 T.....Avocado | 2 T.....Parmesan cheese |
| 1 t.....Butter (2 t whipped) | 1 T.....Pesto (Olive oil) |
| 1 T.....Chocolate, dark (1 oz) | 1 t.....Mayonnaise |
| 1½ T...Coconut milk (⅓ c light) | 1 T.....Salad dressing made |
| 2 T.....Half and Half | with quality oils |
| 8.......Olives, black or green |
| 1 t.....Oils, cooking or salad: Almond, Canola, Coconut (virgin), |
| Grapeseed, Flax Seed Oil (cold pressed), Olive (extra virgin) |
| Safflower or Sunflower high oleic oil, Sesame, Walnut |

*1 serving = 45 calories, 5 g fat*

# Nuts & Seeds

**4** Servings / day □□□□

| | |
|---|---|
| 6.........Almonds | 10.......Peanuts |
| 2.........Brazil nuts | 4.........Pecan halves |
| 6.........Cashews | 1 T.......Pine nuts |
| 3 T......Coconut (unsweetened) | 16.......Pistachios |
| 2 T......Flax seed, ground | 1 T.......Pumpkin seeds |
| 5.........Hazelnuts | 1 T.......Sesame seeds |
| 6.........Mixed nuts (50% | 1 T.......Sunflower seed kernels |
| peanuts) | 2 t.......Tahini (sesame paste) |
| ½ T......Nut butters (1½ t) | 4.........Walnut halves |
| 1 t.......Nut oils |

*1 serving = 45 calories, 5 g fat*

# Protein

**8** Servings / day □□□□□□□□

**Plant Protein:** *(organic, non-GMO preferred)*
1 oz.....Burger alternatives: mushroom, soy, veggie
3 T.......Miso
¼ c.......Natto
1 oz.....Soy foods: soy burgers, soy cheeses, soy dogs
⅓ c.......Tofu, tempeh

**Animal Proteins (very lean cuts or low-fat)**
½ oz.....Beef jerky
1.........Egg or 2 egg whites
½ oz.....Cheese, hard
½ oz.....Cheese, low-fat
¼ c.......Cottage cheese, low-fat

1 oz.....Feta cheese, low-fat
1 oz.....Fish/Shellfish (omega-3 rich: halibut, mackerel, salmon, sardines, tuna)
1 oz.....Meat: beef, buffalo, elk, lamb, pork, veal, venison, wild game
1 oz.....Poultry (skinless chicken, turkey, Cornish hen)
¼ c.......Ricotta cheese, low-fat

**Protein Powder:**
Check label for #grams/scoop
(1 protein serving = 7 g)

*1 oz serving = 50-100 calories, 7 g pro*

# Non-starchy Vegetables

**3-4** Servings / day ■■■■

| | | |
|---|---|---|
| Artichoke | Chard/Swiss Chard | Onions, leeks, shallots |
| Asparagus | Cucumbers | Peppers |
| Bamboo shoots | Eggplant | Radish |
| Bean sprouts | Greens (beet, collard, | Spinach |
| Bell peppers | dandelion, kale, | Squash, summer |
| Bok choy | mustard, turnip) | Tomato |
| Broccoli | Green beans | Vegetable juice (¾ c) |
| Brussels sprouts | Jicama | Fermented vegetables |
| Cabbage | Lettuce | (kimchi, sauerkraut) |
| Carrots | Mushrooms (Crimini, |
| Cauliflower | Shiitake |
| Celery | Okra |

*1 serving = ½ c cooked, 1 c raw, 10 - 25 calories, 5 g carb*

# Core Food Plan

## Enjoy a rainbow of food every day

# Legumes

**2** Servings / day ■■

½ c.....Cooked dried peas, beans, or lentils
¾ c.....Bean soups
½ c.....Edamame, steamed (green soybeans)
⅓ c.....Hummus or other bean dips
½ c.....Fat-free refried beans

*1 serving = 110 calories, 15 g carb, 7 g pro*

# Low-fat Dairy/ Alternatives

**3** Servings / day ■■■

8 oz.....Buttermilk, nonfat or 1%
8 oz.....Kefir, nonfat or 1%
8 oz.....Milks: cow, goat, sheep milk, skim or 1%
8 oz.....Milk alternates: nut, hemp, rice, soy milks; low-fat
6 oz.....Yogurt, cow or soy (plain, nonfat or 1%)
½ c.....Yogurt, Greek (plain, nonfat or 1%)

*1 serving = 70-100 calories, 12 g carb, 7 g pro*

# Starchy Vegetables

**2** Servings / day ■■

| | |
|---|---|
| 1 c.....Acorn squash, cubed | ½ md..Potato (sweet, white) |
| 1 c.....Beets, cubed | ½ c.....Potato, mashed (sweet, |
| 1 c.....Butternut squash, cubed | white) |
| ⅓ c.....Corn | ½ c.....Winter roots or squashes, |
| ½ .......Corn-on-the-cob | (acorn, beet, butternut, |
| ½ c.....Green peas | parsnip, pumpkin, |
| ⅓ c.....Plantain (½ whole) | rutabagas, turnip) |
| 1 c.....Snow peas |

*1 serving = 80 calories, 15 g carb*

# Fruits (No sugar added)

**2** Servings / day ■■

| | |
|---|---|
| 1 sm...Apple | 1 sm...Pear |
| ½ c.....Applesauce | ¾ c.....Pineapple |
| (unsweetened) | 2 sm...Plums |
| 4.........Apricots, fresh | 1 sm...Pomegranate |
| ½ .......Banana, med | 3 md...Prunes |
| ¾ c.....Blackberries | 2 T......Raisins |
| ¾ c.....Blueberries | 1 c.......Raspberries |
| 12.......Cherries | 1¼ c....Strawberries |
| 3.........Dates or Figs | 2 sm...Tangerines |
| ½ c.....Fruit juice | 2 T......Dried fruit |
| ½ ........Grapefruit or | ¼ ........Pear |
| (¾ c sections) |
| 15........Grape | 1 c.......Pineapple |
| 1..........Kiwi |
| ½ sm...Mango |
| 1 sm...Nectarine |
| 1 sm...Orange |
| 1 c.......Papaya |
| 1 sm...Peach |

*1 serving = 60 calories, 15 g carb*

# Grains

**2** Servings / day ■■

| | | |
|---|---|---|
| Amaranth* | Oats | Spelt |
| Bulgur (cracked wheat) | Quinoa* | Tapioca* |
| Buckwheat/kasha* | Rice* | Teff* |
| Kamut | Semolina | Whole wheat |
| Millet* | Sorghum* | *Serving = ⅓-½ c* |

¼.......Bagel, large (whole grain) | ¼ c.....Muesli
⅓ c.....Bulgur, cooked | ⅓ c.....Pasta, whole grain
½ .......Bun (whole grain) | ½ .......Pita, whole grain
1 sl.....Breads, whole grains | 3 c.....Popcorn
½ c.....Cereal, cooked (oatmeal, | ⅓ c.....Quinoa*
wheat, grits) | ½ c.....Rice*
¾ c.....Cereal, ready-to-eat (high | 1 sl.....Rice bread*
fiber, whole grain/rye | 2 .......Rice cakes (brown)*
4-7.....Crackers, whole grain/rye | 3-4.....Rice crackers*
xx........Corn*/Cornmeal* | ⅓ c.....Rice noodles or pasta*
½ c.....Couscous | 1.........Tortilla, 6 inch, whole
½ .......English muffin, whole | grain or rice
grain |
½ c.....Kasha, cooked |

*\* = Gluten free*

*1 serving = 75-110 calories, 15 g carb*

*\* all measurements in single serving sizes*

# CORE DIET, 2,000 CALORIES

## CORE FOOD PLAN

### DAILY FOOD INTAKE

### DAILY FLUID INTAKE

½ **of your desirable weight (lbs) in ounces**
**Best Choice:** Purified water
**Other Options:**
Unsweetened beverages low in
salt/sodium and caffeine

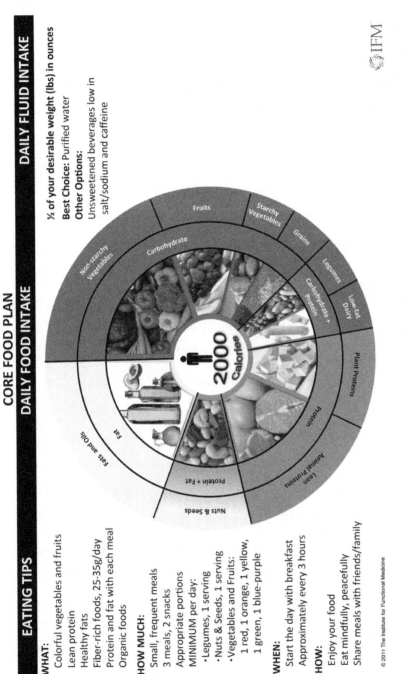

### EATING TIPS

**WHAT:**
Colorful vegetables and fruits
Lean protein
Healthy fats
Fiber-rich foods, 25-35g/day
Protein and fat with each meal
Organic foods

**HOW MUCH:**
Small, frequent meals
3 meals, 2 snacks
Appropriate portions
MINIMUM per day:
· Legumes, 1 serving
· Nuts & Seeds, 1 serving
· Vegetables and Fruits:
  1 red, 1 orange, 1 yellow,
  1 green, 1 blue-purple

**WHEN:**
Start the day with breakfast
Approximately every 3 hours

**HOW:**
Enjoy your food
Eat mindfully, peacefully
Share meals with friends/family

© 2011 The Institute for Functional Medicine

## Fats & Oils

9 Servings / day

2 T.....Avocado
1 t......Butter (2 t. whipped)
1 T.....Chocolate, dark (1 oz)
1½ T..Coconut milk (⅓ c light)
2 T ...Half and Half
8........Olives, black or green
1 t......Oils, cooking or salad: Almond, Canola, Coconut (virgin), Grapeseed, Flax Seed Oil (cold pressed), Olive (extra virgin) Safflower or Sunflower high oleic oil, Sesame, Walnut
2 T.....Parmesan cheese
1 T.....Pesto (Olive oil)
1 t......Mayonnaise
1 T.....Salad dressing made with quality oils

*1 serving = 45 calories, 5 g fat*

## Nuts & Seeds

4 Servings / day

6........Almonds
2........Brazil nuts
6........Cashews
3 T.....Coconut (unsweetened)
2 T.....Flax seed, ground
5........Hazelnuts
6........Mixed nuts (50% peanuts)
½ T....Nut butters (1½ t)
1 t......Nut oils
10......Peanuts
4........Pecan halves
1 T.....Pine nuts
16......Pistachios
1 T.....Pumpkin seeds
1 T.....Sesame seeds
1 T.....Sunflower seed kernels
2 t......Tahini (sesame paste)
4........Walnut halves

*1 serving = 45 calories, 5 g fat*

## Protein

10 Servings / day

**Plant Protein:** (*organic, non-GMO preferred*)
1 oz...Burger alternatives: mushroom, soy, veggie
3 T.....Miso
¼ c....Natto
1 oz...Soy foods: soy burgers, soy cheeses, soy dogs
½ c....Tofu, tempeh

**Animal Proteins (very lean cuts or low-fat)**
½ oz..Beef jerky
1........Egg or 2 egg whites
½ oz..Cheese, hard
1 oz...Cheese, low-fat
¼ c....Cottage cheese, low-fat
1 oz...Feta cheese, low-fat
1 oz...Fish/Shellfish (omega-3 rich: halibut, mackerel, salmon, sardines, tuna)
1 oz...Meat: beef, buffalo, elk, lamb, pork, veal, venison, wild game
1 oz...Poultry (skinless chicken, turkey, Cornish hen)
¼ c....Ricotta cheese, low-fat

**Protein Powder:**
Check label for #grams/scoop (1 protein serving = 7 g)

*1 oz serving = 50-100 calories, 7 g pro*

* all measurements in single serving sizes

## Non-starchy Vegetables

5 Servings / day

Artichoke
Asparagus
Bamboo shoots
Bean sprouts
Bell peppers
Bok choy
Broccoli
Brussels sprouts
Cabbage
Carrots
Cauliflower
Celery
Chard/Swiss Chard
Cucumbers
Eggplant
Greens (beet, collard, dandelion, kale, mustard, turnip)
Green beans
Jicama
Lettuce
Mushrooms (Crimini, Shiitake
Okra
Onions, leeks, shallots
Peppers
Radish
Spinach
Squash, summer
Tomato
Vegetable juice (¾ c)
Fermented vegetables (kimchi, sauerkraut)

*1 serving = ½ c cooked, 1 c raw, 10- 25 calories, 5 g carb*

# Core Food Plan

**Enjoy a rainbow of food every day**

## Legumes

3 Servings / day

½ c....Cooked dried peas, beans, or lentils
¾ c....Bean soups
½ c....Edamame, steamed (green soybeans)
⅓ c....Hummus or other bean dips
½ c....Fat-free refried beans

*1 serving = 110 calories, 15 g carb, 7 g pro*

## Low-fat Dairy/ Alternatives

3 Servings / day

8 oz...Buttermilk, nonfat or 1%
8 oz...Kefir, nonfat or 1%
8 oz...Milks: cow, goat, sheep milk, skim or 1%
8 oz...Milk alternates: nut, hemp, rice, soy milks; low-fat
6 oz...Yogurt, cow or soy (plain, nonfat or 1%)
½ c....Yogurt, Greek (plain, nonfat or 1%)

*1 serving = 70-100 calories, 12 g carb, 7 g pro*

## Starchy Vegetables

2 Servings / day

1 c.....Acorn squash, cubed
1 c.....Beets, cubed
1 c.....Butternut squash, cubed
½ c....Corn
½ ......Corn-on-the-cob
½ c....Green peas
⅓ c....Plantain (½ whole)
1 c.....Snow peas
½ md.Potato (sweet, white)
½ c....Potato, mashed (sweet, white)
½ c...Winter roots or squashes, (acorn, beet, butternut, parsnip, pumpkin, rutabagas, turnip)

*1 serving = 80 calories, 15 g carb*

## Fruits (No sugar added)

3 Servings / day

1 sm .Apple
½ c. ...Applesauce (unsweetened)
4........Apricots, fresh
½.......Banana, med
¾ c....Blackberries
¾ c....Blueberries
12......Cherries
3........Dates or Figs
½ c....Fruit juice
½.......Grapefruit or (¾ c sections)
15......Grape
1........Kiwi
½ sm.Mango
1 c.....Melon
1 sm..Nectarine
1 sm..Orange
1 c.....Papaya
1 sm..Peach
1 sm..Pear
¾ c....Pineapple
2 sm..Plums
1 sm..Pomegranate
3 md .Prunes
2 T.....Raisins
1 c.....Raspberries
1¼ c..Strawberries
2 sm..Tangerines
2 T.....Dried fruit

*1 serving = 60 calories, 15 g carb*

## Grains

3 Servings / day

Amaranth*
Bulgur (cracked wheat)
Buckwheat/kasha*
Kamut
Millet*
Oats
Quinoa*
Rice*
Semolina
Sorghum*
Spelt
Tapioca*
Teff*
Whole wheat

*Serving = ⅓-½ c*

¼.......Bagel, large (whole grain)
½ c....Bulgur, cooked
½.......Bun (whole grain)
1 sl ....Breads, whole grains
½ c....Cereal, cooked (oatmeal, wheat, grits)
¾ c....Cereal, ready-to-eat (high fiber, whole grain)
4-7.....Crackers, whole grain/rye
xx......Corn*/Cornmeal*
⅓ c....Couscous
½ ......English muffin, whole grain
½ c....Kasha, cooked
¼ c....Muesli
⅓ c....Pasta, whole grain
½.......Pita, whole grain
3 c.....Popcorn
⅓ c....Quinoa*
⅓ c....Rice*
1 sl. ...Rice bread*
2 .......Rice cakes (brown)*
3-4.....Rice crackers*
⅓ c....Rice noodles or pasta*
1........Tortilla, 6 inch, whole grain or rice

* = Gluten free

*1 serving = 75-110 calories, 15 g carb*

# PATIENT PHYTONUTRIENT HANDOUT

## Eat a Rainbow of Healthy Foods

### GREEN

**Foods**

| | | |
|---|---|---|
| Apples | Brussels sprouts | collard, dandelion, kale, lettuce, mustard, spinach, turnip) |
| Artichoke | Cabbage | |
| Asparagus | Celery | Limes |
| Avocado | Cucumbers | Okra |
| Bamboo sprouts | Edamame/Soy beans | Olives |
| Bean sprouts | Green beans | Pears |
| Bell Peppers | Green peas | Rosemary |
| Bitter melon | Green tea | Snow peas |
| Bok choy | Greens (beet, chard/swiss chard, | Watercress |
| Broccoli | | |
| Broccolini | | |

**Benefits**

- Anti-cancer
- Anti-inflammatory
- Brain health
- Cell protection
- Skin health
- Hormone balance
- Heart health
- Liver health

### YELLOW

**Foods**

| | | |
|---|---|---|
| Apple (Golden Delicious) | Corn-on-the-cob | Pineapple |
| Asian pears | Ginger root | Potatoes (Yukon) |
| Banana | Greens | Spinach |
| Bell peppers | Kale | Starfruit |
| Corn | Lemon | Succotash |

**Benefits**

- Anti-cancer
- Anti-inflammatory
- Cell protection
- Cognition
- Eye health
- Heart health
- Skin health
- Vascular health

### ORANGE

**Foods**

| | | |
|---|---|---|
| Acorn squash | Dried fruit (apricot, mango, papaya) | Persimmons |
| Apricots | | Pumpkin |
| Bell pepper | Mango | Sweet potato |
| Butternut squash | Nectarine | Tangerines |
| Cantaloupe | Orange | Tea (orange infused) |
| Carrots | Papaya | Turmeric root |

**Benefits**

- Anti-cancer
- Anti-bacterial
- Immune health
- Cell protection
- Reduced mortality
- Reproductive health
- Skin health
- Source of vitamin A

### RED

**Foods**

| | | |
|---|---|---|
| Adzuki beans | Grapes | Raspberries |
| Apples | Kidney beans | Shrimp |
| Applesauce | Onions | Strawberries |
| Bell Peppers | Plums | Sweet red peppers |
| Cranberries | Pomegranate | Rhubarb |
| Cherries | Potatoes | Rooibos tea |
| Grapefruit (pink) | Radicchio | Tomato |
| Goji berries | Radishes | |

**Benefits**

- Anti-cancer
- Anti-inflammatory
- Cell protection
- DNA health
- Immune health
- Prostate health
- Vascular health

### BLUE/PURPLE

**Foods**

| | | |
|---|---|---|
| Bell pepper | Carrots | Plums |
| Berries (blue, black, boysenberries, huckleberries, marionberries) | Cauliflower | Potatoes |
| | Eggplant | Prunes |
| | Figs | Raisins |
| | Grapes | Rice, (black or purple) |
| Cabbage | Kale | |
| | Olives | |

**Benefits**

- Anti-cancer
- Anti-inflammatory
- Cell protection
- Cognitive health
- Heart health
- Liver health

### WHITE/TAN

**Foods**

| | | |
|---|---|---|
| Apples | Garlic | Refried beans |
| Bean dips | Legumes (hummus, dried beans or peas, lentils, chickpeas, peanuts) | (low-fat) |
| Cauliflower | | Sauerkraut |
| Cinnamon | | Sesame seeds |
| Clove | | Shallots |
| Coconut products | Lychee | Soy |
| Coffee | Mushrooms | Tahini |
| Dark chocolate | Nuts | Tea (black, white) |
| Dates | Onions | Whole flaxseeds |
| Flaxseed meal | Pears | Whole grains |

**Benefits**

- Anti-cancer
- Anti-inflammatory
- Cell protection
- Gastrointestinal health
- Heart health
- Hormone health
- Liver health

IFM

# SUPPLEMENT GUIDE

**1. UltraInflamX**, by Metagenics: This medical food has a low allergy potential protein base with anti-inflammatory herbs and extra nutrients that help with detoxification.

**Recommended use:** Start with half a scoop and work up to two scoops two times a day. Mix the powder into water or any juice that's allowable on the elimination diet.

**What to expect:** Generally, people tolerate this very well. The most common side effect is gas and bloating because of the fiber, which is why I recommend working up to the full dosage. If you are allergic to one of the ingredients, don't use this product.

**2. IgG 2000** by Xymogen: The technical term for this product is serum-derived bovine immunoglobulins. This powder contains powerful immune components from the blood of an organic herd of cattle in Iowa. IgG 2000 is similar to colostrum but has much higher levels of the immune components than colostrum has. Cows have probiotic species in their gut that are similar to ours, and they don't make antibodies against their own probiotic bacteria. Conversely, they're under attack by a wide variety of pathogens and potential pathogens that they *do* make antibodies against. So the powder has antibodies against a wide variety of bacteria, viruses, and fungus but no immune activity against the good bacteria. It differs from antibiotics, which kill everything. In this case, it's more of a smart bomb that will kill off the bad guys and preserve the good guys.

**Recommended use:** Take a tablespoon of this powder twice a day. The powder is slightly oily because of an oil used in the extraction process, so the best way to consume it is to mix it into the dry UltraInflamX, then add the fluid and shake vigorously.

**What to expect:** With the IgG 2000, we're waging biological warfare in the gut; in other words, we're killing off bad bugs, which are not going to be happy about that. They'll defend themselves by revving up metabolism and producing more gas, so gas and bloating is common. However, this is not because of the IgG 2000; it's the bad bugs in the gut that haven't yet figured out that resistance is futile. If symptoms become severe or overwhelming, stop and restart at a lower dose.

**3. ProbioMax** by Xymogen: This is a potent probiotic containing 100 billion bacteria per pill. These are good guys. We're using the IgG 2000 to get rid of the bad guys, the UltraInflamX to reduce inflammation and give nutrients to heal the gut, and ProbioMax will give your gut healthy bacteria that should result in a healthier immune system and healthier gut lining. When you go to the health food store, you'll generally find a probiotic that contains between three and six billion bacteria per bill. If you search hard, you'll find 20 or 60 billion. This is 100 billion. Isn't this too much? No. There are 100 *trillion* bacteria in your gut already, so the dose is tantamount to spitting in the ocean.

**Recommended use:** Take one pill twice a day.

**What to expect:** If you have advanced liver disease or a severely injured colon from ischemic bowel disease, you shouldn't take this without a physician's advice. Otherwise, this product will have similar side effects as the previous supplements: we're reinforcing the army of the probiotic species in your gut, and the dysbiotic species won't be happy about it. They'll rev up metabolism and make gas. Fortunately, the UltraInflamX will mitigate some of this biological warfare by reducing inflammation.

**4. EPA/DHA 720** by Metagenics: This concentrated form of fish oil provides anti-inflammatory properties to help heal the gut. In natural medicine, we alter a number of pathways in a synergistic way, so the EPA/DHA will reduce inflammation in a different way than the previous supplements by competing for the same enzyme that converts arachidonic acid (a polyunsaturated omega-6 fatty acid) to pro-inflammatory cytokines. At the same time, the fish oil feeds anti-inflammatory pathways.

**Recommended use:** Two pills twice a day gives a therapeutic anti-inflammatory dose.

**What to expect:** EPA/DHA 720 is generally recognized as safe for healthy adults. If you use blood-thinners or have other coagulopathies or bleeding disorders, consult with your doctor before beginning use. Typically, the biggest side effect to fish oil is burping fish. The best way to manage that is to keep the fish oil in the freezer and take it frozen, because it will get further into your digestive system before it melts and opens up.

**5. Dynamic Greens** by Nutrition Dynamics: Dynamic greens are carefully selected fruit and vegetable powders with known anti-inflammatory and detoxification properties. Each scoop has the antioxidant capacity of 20 servings of fruits and veggies.

**Recommended use:** Take one scoop twice a day. If you mix it dry with the UltraInflamX and IgG 2000 before pouring fluid, it will combine smoothly instead of clumping.

**What to expect:** With the exception of having an allergy to one of the constituents of Dynamic Greens, this supplement is generally very well tolerated.

All of these supplements can be ordered through a healthcare professional or through http://3rdopinion.us.

⊙-⊙-⊙

Remember, if you are not seeing progress with the suggestions in this book, it should not be taken as a sign that functional medicine does not work. Instead, it should be taken as a sign that your case requires a more thorough examination by a skilled and practiced functional medicine practitioner with access to the wide range of individualized nutritional biochemical interventions.

**Just be well!**

CPSIA information can be obtained
at www.ICGtesting.com
Printed in the USA
BVOW06s0101080817
491447BV00008B/96/P